PLAN·D™
cookbook
FLOURLESS & SUGARLESS CUISINE

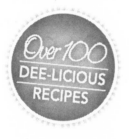

Over 100 DEE-LICIOUS RECIPES

DEE MCCAFFREY, CDC

CENTER
FOR PROCESSED-FREE
LIVING
PUBLISHING

All proceeds from the sale of this book go directly to the Center for Processed-Free Living

Plan-D Cookbook: Flourless and Sugarless Cuisine
By Dee McCaffrey

This is a unique and revised edition of <u>Dee's Mighty Cookbook: Tasty Cuisine for Flourless and Sugarless Living</u>

Printed in the United States of America.

Cover Design: Jennifer Rose
Cover Photograph: Paul Markow

The Center for Processed-Free Living
P.O. Box 27564
Tempe, AZ 85285-7564

ISBN: 978-0-9745530-5-4

Table of Contents

Acknowledgements

There are some special people that I must thank for helping make this book possible: Jennifer Dally for diligently transcribing the scraps of paper I called my recipes; Bob Cash for his patient proofreading and editing; and Ed Barker for his kind guidance and invaluable support. All my friends and students, for your contribution to this book, both with your recipes and your encouragement to complete this project. My mother Carol, for her humble example of the importance of self-empowerment through an education. Finally, a special thanks goes to my partner and husband, Michael, without whom all this would not be possible. I am truly grateful for all that you bring into my life and into my heart.

Thank you all for being so special in my life and for your unwavering support.

Introduction

Dear Mindful Eaters:

One of the first things my nutrition students learn is that foods made with refined sugar and white flour are the bane of weight loss and good health. The second thing they learn is that we can live "flourless" and "sugarless" and still enjoy life. In the past 50-100 years, our food supply has changed dramatically. We have gone from growing, harvesting, and preparing our own food with our own hands, to mass-producing concoctions that are made in food laboratories. Refined sugar, white flour, artificial sweeteners, trans-fats, chemical preservatives, flavor enhancers, and stabilizers have replaced the real foods that our not-so-distant ancestors ate. We've become so far removed from foods in their natural state, that we now call them "health foods," a sad admission that we've compromised our health for the sake of convenience.

The importance of "flourless and sugarless living" is clear from my experience and that of many others. Refined sugars and flours rob the human body of many essential vitamins and minerals, and in many cases are the main cause of obesity. After myriad attempts and failures at losing weight, I was fortunate in the early 1990's to become affiliated with a support group where a small faction of members were refraining from eating all forms of sugar and flour. This at first seemed difficult to do, but I saw success in those who had been living sugar and flour-free for many years. People who had struggled their entire lives with obesity, now lived in normal-sized bodies—some of them 150 to 200 pounds lighter—without desire or pangs of deprivation for the starchy sugar-laden foods we had all grown up eating. Seasoned members claimed that sugar and flour were addictive substances, which when eaten on a regular basis, caused cravings that led to overeating. More than that, many of them claimed that their migraine headaches, arthritis, and diabetes had vanished after giving up flour and sugar. With trepidation, I decided to give it a try. In April of 1992, I eliminated all forms of refined sugar and flour from my life. The result was a 100 pound weight loss that I have sustained for over 14 years.

Before, during, and after my weight loss, I spent many years working as a chemist in a laboratory. My 100 pound weight loss served as the impetus for learning the "how's" and "why's" of proper nutrition. In 2000, I attended Bauman College to broaden my education in nutrition. My chemistry background became invaluable as I learned the truth about how sugar, fats, and carbohydrates affect body chemistry and speed up the degradation of our bodies. In this book, I share with you, in layman's terms, why these foods are so harmful. You will also discover the six most important foods for weight loss and good health.

My definition of "flourless" describes foods that do not contain any flours that have been through a refinement process. The refinement process strips apart a whole grain to remove its fiber and bleaches out nutrients in order to extend the shelf-life of the resulting flour. Refined flours come under the following names: wheat flour, bleached flour, unbleached wheat flour, enriched flour, unbleached enriched wheat flour, 100% wheat flour, multigrain, rye flour, and pumpernickel among others. Whole grain flours—which are flours that consist of the entire grain— retaining all fiber and nutrients—are included in some of the recipes. These include 100% whole wheat, spelt, and oat flours. Whole grain flours have a shorter shelf-life, but they contain all of the fiber and nutrients necessary for longevity and good health. It is a mystery science has not been able to explain, but it's true. Walter Willett, Ph.D., chair of the nutrition department at the Harvard School of Public Health, explains that all foods found in nature, when eaten in their natural whole state, contain all the corresponding fiber, nutrients, and enzymes the human body requires to properly digest that particular food. When we eat manipulated foods like flour, sugar, and artificial ingredients, we're eating something the body doesn't recognize as food. They cannot be properly digested, causing problems for our health down the road.

"Sugarless" refers to foods that are free of refined sugars. Sugar cane, beets, and corn undergo similar refining and bleaching processes to wheat—removing pulp, fiber, enzymes, vitamins, and minerals—resulting in a nutritionally empty form of sugar. These forms include white sugar, light and dark brown sugar, raw sugar, corn syrup, high fructose corn syrup, molasses, beet sugar, most commercial honey, refined fruit juices, dextrose, sucrose, fructose, glucose, and maltose. Naturally-sweet foods— which are brimming with fiber and nutrients—are included in some of the recipes. These include organic unrefined raw honey, organic pure maple syrup, and *Rapadura*, a form of organically grown unrefined sugar cane. For those who want to eliminate even natural sweeteners, there is a very healthy natural herbal sweetener called stevia, which is not a sugar at all. I go into great detail about stevia in the chapter "The Six Most Important Foods for Weight Loss and Good Health."

The recipes contained in this book allow you to get back in touch with the life-giving qualities of food. Go forth, enjoy, and be healthy!

7

A Special Note to Diabetics

Some of the recipes in this book call for natural sweeteners that are not appropriate for diabetics to consume. Although raw unfiltered honey, pure maple syrup and Rapadura contain valuable fiber, enzymes and nutrients; the natural sugars contained in them can exacerbate a diabetic condition. The preferred sweetener for anyone who is diabetic, and the ONLY sweetener I recommend, is *stevia* (see index). This natural sweetener does not affect blood sugar levels and is, therefore, safe for diabetic consumption. Even if you are not diabetic, you would do well to replace sugar with this healthy alternative. Artificial sweeteners such as saccharine (Sweet 'n Low), Aspartame (Nutrasweet and Equal), Acesulfame Potassium (Acesulfame K), and Sucralose (Splenda) should be avoided due to their unnatural chemical properties, which have been linked to many health conditions and diseases.

A Special Note to Celiacs

My definition of "flourless" refers to foods that do not contain any flours that have been through a refinement process. If you are intolerant to wheat and/or gluten, the majority of the recipes in this book are safe for you to eat. Only four of them call for whole wheat flour and a few others recommend flourless sprouted grain bread. Sprouted grain breads that contain gluten can be substituted with any gluten-free bread.

There are a number of gluten-free flours that can be substituted for whole wheat, such as amaranth, spelt, quinoa, brown rice and buckwheat (buckwheat is not a wheat), however the textures of the recipes may be different and so the amounts may have to be altered.

My Story

My mother tells me that when I was a little girl, people used to ask her if she was feeding me enough because I was so thin, but I don't remember a time when I wasn't overeating and overweight. I started gaining weight at the age of nine, and I was overweight until the age of 31. That was the year my parents divorced, and I began eating to avoid feeling conflict, comforting my fears, and suppressing anger over a situation with which I had no control. My trip to the corner store after school to buy candy was the highlight of my day. I remember sneaking slices of bread or chunks of salami and hiding in my room to eat them. Eating made me forget about the emptiness I felt when my father left, and unconsciously food became my principal source of happiness.

As early as fifth grade, I refused to wear dresses to school because I didn't want the boys to make fun of my fat legs. In high school, despite playing on the tennis team (which I was good at and really wanted to do), I continued to gain weight. Those were especially painful years, as I became more aware of what I was missing out on because of my weight. I never had a boyfriend and didn't attend my proms. I was quiet and shy and ashamed of my weight, so I related to food and books instead of my classmates. After graduation, I moved out on my own, and it was then that my eating and weight began to soar. By the time I was eighteen, I weighed 180 pounds.

As a young adult, it was baffling to me why I ate like there was no tomorrow. I had done it all my life and didn't know any other way. And sugary foods—donuts, pastries, cookies, candy bars, mint chocolate chip ice cream and anything else chocolate—these were the foods I loved the most. Also, I couldn't resist crunchy salty snacks like corn chips, potato chips, and popcorn. My meals were high in starch, sugar and fat. Bread, pizza, salami sandwiches, spaghetti, macaroni & cheese, and Dr. Pepper were staples throughout my 20's. Nary a vegetable or a piece of fruit passed my lips. Peanut m&m's were my favorite. I could inhale a whole one-pound bag in an evening.

My first attempt to lose weight began at the age of nineteen—the beginning of a series of failed attempts. My story is typical—I never lost enough to reach a healthy goal weight, and I always gained back more than I lost. By my late 20's I finally gave up trying to diet and my weight hovered steadily over 200 pounds. I'm 4'10" with a petite body frame, so that's twice the weight of what someone my size should weigh!

One day in February of 1992, overstuffed from a super-sized lunch, I ransacked the cupboards looking for something more to eat. I found some old, stale candy from the previous Halloween that I didn't even like. As I sat on my couch eating this disgusting candy, it occurred to me that something was seriously wrong with me. In that moment, I had a vision of myself as an old woman nearing the end of my days wishing for a life that could have been. I saw that I had been an observer standing on the sidelines watching my life go by and not participating in it.

For as long as I could remember, I had let my weight hold me back from being my true self and pursuing the things in life that I knew would make me happy. I was so afraid of people, yet inside I longed for intimacy and friendship. I was shy, quiet, and ashamed of my weight. I did not actively seek out people as friends because I felt that no one would like me because I was fat. My obesity stripped me of my self-esteem, talked me out of taking risks, imprisoned me in isolation, and robbed me of my identity. The fat kept me from believing in myself and diminished my spirit. I felt trapped by my weight and I was in a state of hopeless despair.

Nothing about my life changed that day, but a month later I had what can only be described as a profound inner change. I reached an epiphany and "the day came when the desire to remain the same was more painful than the risk to grow." I was on a field trip in college that involved hiking up a very steep hill. For some reason I thought it would be easy, never mind the fact that I smoked a pack of cigarettes every day, and by this time I was at my top weight, which had climbed to somewhere over 210 pounds. It was more than a struggle to pull my fat body up that hill. My legs were hurting, my heart was pounding, and I could hardly breathe. I was filled with shame and humiliation when I realized how out of shape my body was and that I could not keep up with the other people. I felt as though they were all looking at me, waiting for the fat girl to get to the top. Then I was afraid I was going to die, if not on the side of that hill, then soon.

Miraculously, I made it to the top. I walked over to join the rest of the class and when I got there, my foot slipped out from under me and I fell flat on my rear. I was filled with humiliation and embarrassment, and I turned my head and looked away from the crowd. At the top of the hill, looking out over the beautiful San Francisco Bay, I felt like the lowest thing on earth. Suddenly, a wave of realization overcame me. It stripped denial from me; life stood starkly in front of me, demanding my attention. I looked at it for what seemed like a long time and I wanted to cry. The physical condition of my body was symbolic of how I had let everything in my life get out of control. *I* had let this happen. I was horrified.

11

When I returned home from the hiking trip, I deadened my pain by once again eating myself into oblivion. Each time I relived the hiking trip in my mind, I heard a voice coming from somewhere deep inside me. The message was loud and clear: CHANGE YOUR LIFE OR DIE. Those words frightened me and I turned to the only method I had ever known to cope with fear—I ate. And I continued to eat until the pain of overeating was worse than the thought of having to change my life.

Then on April 3rd, 1992, something shifted inside me. I cannot describe how I got there, but I finally gave up the struggle. Instead of dieting, I started learning and living. I began to believe in myself and became committed to making my dream of losing my excess weight come true. For the first time in my life, I took responsibility and became accountable to myself by measuring my food at every meal and keeping a record of everything I ate and how I was feeling.

I began to educate myself on nutrition. I read, with enthusiasm and vigor, book after book on nutrition, body chemistry, food combining, metabolism and more. From all of this reading and with the help of my organic chemistry background, I developed my own healthy eating plan and followed it like my life depended on it. I stopped eating all of the foods that had historically been problems for me. These included anything made with sugar and refined carbohydrates, fatty foods, processed foods, fried foods, alcohol, and caffeine. I started eating things I never liked before, such as fresh vegetables and fruits, unrefined whole grains, lean poultry and fish. I never felt so much freedom around food before in my life. It seemed ironic, but once I introduced discipline into my food choices, I was free to enjoy eating rather than being a slave to it. Because

12

there was structure and discipline around my eating, I was able to put food in its proper perspective.

Although I enjoy my meals, now I eat them to nurture my body and spirit, not in response to my emotional fluctuations of the day. Planning my meals ahead of time allowed me to learn how to separate food from feelings. The eating plan became my anchor—the one steady constant in my quickly changing life.

Walking became my mode of transportation on the road to healthy living. I started with slow and short walks, and rapidly worked my way up to brisk, aerobic 60 minute walks. I took my walks alone because I used the time not only for exercise, but also for contemplative thinking. Walking helped to build and strengthen my body as well as to build and strengthen my relationship with myself. It gave me the spiritual nourishment and energy to change and reshape my life. As the days, weeks, and months passed, I watched my shadow get smaller and smaller, and my spirit grow larger and larger.

Another discipline instrumental to my weight loss was the practice of writing and journaling. This enabled me to identify the emotions that were associated with my eating. I learned that the discomfort I felt when dieting, that sense of deprivation, was not about food and never had been. I had to write to find out what in my life was so painfully absent and what certain foods represented in my emotional life. For instance, one time after I binged on a big bag of popcorn, a good friend suggested that I write down everything I could remember about eating popcorn. It was through this exercise that I was able to identify my emotional attachment to popcorn.

When I was a little girl my mother used to make enough popcorn to fill a grocery bag when our family sat together to watch television. Mom was always happy, and when mom was happy, the mood in the room was loving and safe. At a young age, I associated that big bag of popcorn with mom being happy and the family being close. Several years later after my mom and dad had divorced, there was tremendous pain in the family.

During my troubled teen years, I only knew that eating popcorn gave me a good feeling, and I had subconsciously disassociated from the original emotional ties that had initiated those good feelings. The taste and smell of popcorn went straight to my heart, so whenever I was around it, I immediately wanted to eat it. When I dieted and didn't allow myself to eat popcorn, I felt *so* deprived. Eventually, and without fail, I would then binge on huge amounts of popcorn. In reality, I was looking to recapture the love and closeness from those days of old. That was what was truly missing in my life, not popcorn. From then on, whenever I craved a particular food, I did this particular writing exercise to help break the emotional attachment. Over time, although slowly, I was able to free myself from these attachments. One by one, I worked hard to identify my weaknesses and erase the conditioning that trapped me for so long.

It took me a little more than a year to lose the 100 pounds of excess weight. I went from a size 22 to a size 4! I realized two of my lifelong dreams simultaneously. First I finally reached my goal weight, 108 pounds. Second, I graduated from college, the first female on my mother's side of the family, and the first ever on my father's side. Both of these dreams were such milestones, because I never believed that either one of them would come true. I did not begin college until the age of twenty-six, and it wasn't until my last two semesters, while I was in the process of losing the weight and changing my life, that I was able to focus and excel in my course work.

The unwavering belief in myself, the commitment to a daily eating and exercise regimen, the release of those awful emotional attachments, and a deep sense of wholeness gave me confidence, self-esteem, and a freedom from shame and humiliation. Even over a decade later, it is still a conscious choice to eat healthy food and exercise every day. I still write out my feelings, and I continue to work on my personal growth. My life before losing weight was all about unfulfilled desires. I wanted to perform and dance and sing; I wanted to have a wealth of friends and acquaintances; I wanted a fulfilling profession; and most of all, I wanted to be comfortable just being in my skin.

Over the years, I have achieved all of those things and so much more. I have come into my own, reclaiming and enhancing my true self that was buried so deeply for so many years. There have been many ups and downs in my life, and I have not succumbed to finding comfort, celebration, or relief in excess food. I endured the pain and devastation of divorce from my first husband, financial scarcity, three major moves, a serious illness that left me hospitalized, two miscarriages, and four family deaths. I also relished in the excitement of dating in my new body, falling head over heals in love, and marrying the man of my dreams. I have witnessed the wonderment and awe as my creative talents and abilities completely came to life. From writing poetry to singing and performing in community theater, from leading and facilitating workshops to writing and directing plays, I am now living the life I had only dreamed of. And I have come to know the deep connection of true friendship and intimacy and now feel worthy of it. I've learned that there is wisdom, friendship, and profit in just being real; that who I am is good enough and the whole world is invited to see and connect with me.

Now, I feel a deep sense of responsibility to bring hope to others who suffer as I once did. Early in my weight loss process, I discovered that I have a passion for helping others with their own weight and food issues. This passion eventually led me to broaden my education in holistic nutrition, and drove me to expand my professional work as an organic chemist to include being a nutrition and weight loss counselor. I now teach nutrition and weight loss classes and provide one-on-one diet counseling. My intention is to create a space for change, to educate and enlighten others on the value of holistic nutrition, and to support them in their transition to healthy living.

What started in my early years as a hollow desire to be thin has become so much more than I would have ever prayed for on that fateful day overlooking the San Francisco Bay. Although I would never wish it on anyone else, I'm grateful for my experience as an overweight person. It has given me compassion for others, it's kept me mindful of where I could be again, and it's allowed me to more fully appreciate my life and my relationships with others.

Outside the walking and the mental tools that I developed, the recipes in this book helped change my life. Over time, my students added great new recipes I now enjoy, and I appreciate their love and support.

So, don't give up. If I can lose half my weight and keep it off to this day for over a decade, you can too. Read on, stay committed, and enjoy the beautiful life you have and the even more beautiful life that is yet to come.

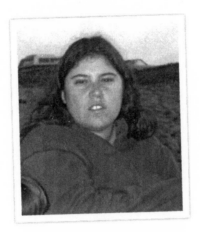

Summer 1984

What should have been a cool day
at the beach was clouded by the
unhappiness in my life. At age 23,
I weighed over 200 pounds.

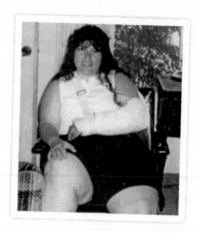

July 1990

Here I am in all my glory, just
after my honeymoon at age 29. My
weight had climbed to over 210
pounds, and I was still gaining.

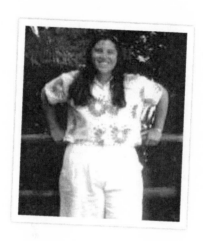

July 1992

Three and a half months after
giving up flour and sugar, I had
lost 48 pounds. At 162 pounds, I
felt light and happy.

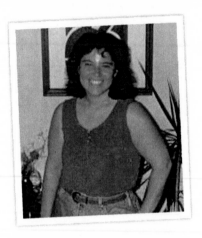

August 1992

It's amazing how quickly the
weight came off after giving up
flour and sugar. After four and a
half months, I had lost 61 pounds
and was still going strong. I was
149 ½ pounds in this picture.

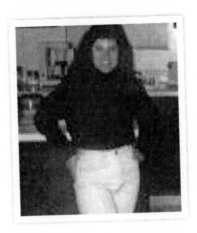

January 1993

The weight came off more slowly
as I got thinner. After 9 and a
half months of staying away
from flour and sugar, I had lost
92 pounds. Almost at my goal
weight, I weighed 118 pounds.

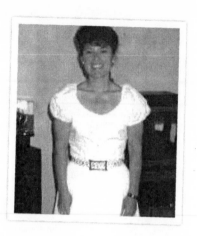

May 1993

My dreams have come true. Here
I am on the day I graduated from
college and one full year after staying
away from flour and sugar. I lost 102
pounds and weighed 108 pounds. By
staying away from flour and sugar and
anything artificial, I have maintained
this weight for over a decade.

What's so Bad About Flour and Sugar?

The initial reason for eliminating flour and sugar from my diet was the strong personal evidence that I was addicted to the stuff. Many books have been written on the subject of food addiction, all of them subscribing to the theory that refined carbohydrates are addictive due to their refined nature. Being a scientist, I needed a more compelling reason.

The United States is facing a health crisis unlike anything seen in human history. Today, fully 65 percent of American adults are overweight, and nearly half of them can be classified as obese. Among children between the ages of 6 and 19 years old, 15 percent—or one in six—are overweight. Another 15 percent are on their way to obesity.

Obesity is second only to lung cancer as the leading cause of preventable death. Furthermore, the number of people suffering from diabetes, arthritis, osteoporosis, cancer, and heart disease—all diet related illnesses—is staggering.

Obesity and most of today's common health problems were rare 100 years ago when people's diets consisted of stone-ground whole grains and high fiber foods. And contrary to the thoughts surrounding the low-carb craze, all carbohydrates are not the problem. The problem is the *type* of carbohydrate.

Our bodies absolutely need carbohydrates, as they provide most of the energy we require to work, exercise, and play. The brain's preferred fuel comes from the glucose provided by the breakdown of carbohydrates in our bodies. There are two natural forms of carbohydrates, simple and complex. Then there is the "refined" carbohydrate.

Simple carbohydrates are quickly digested, enabling the body to absorb the glucose necessary to provide short energy bursts. Examples of simple carbohydrates are fruits, fruit juices, honey, molasses, pure maple syrup, and sugar.

Complex carbohydrates take longer to digest, the resulting glucose being more slowly absorbed into the body and providing energy over a longer period of time. Examples of complex carbohydrates are fresh vegetables, beans and peas, and whole grains—such as oats, barley, brown rice, rye, and whole wheat. Complex carbohydrates contain an abundance of vitamins and minerals that are vital to health. They are also very high in fiber. Whole grains contain bran and germ, two important fibers. Fiber is important because it helps the body to process waste efficiently and helps us to feel fuller for longer.

A "refined" carbohydrate is a carbohydrate that has been altered by machinery to increase its shelf-life. The refinement process transforms a complex carbohydrate into a simple carbohydrate by removing the original natural elements such as fiber, healthy oils, vitamins, and minerals.

Relying heavily on commercial food products, the American diet is rife with the refined carbohydrates found in white sugar, white rice and white flour.

Examples include breads, crackers, pastries, baked goods, pastas, most commercial cereals, ice cream, chocolates, pizza, sandwiches, fast foods and snack foods of all types. These products are so highly refined that the body doesn't even recognize them as food.

Although most people don't understand their bodies' nutritional requirements, their bodies themselves do. All foods found in nature, when eaten in their natural whole state, contain the corresponding nutrients and enzymes the

24

body requires to properly digest that particular food. It's a mystery science has not been able to explain, but it's true. Fruits, legumes, whole grains, vegetables, and even raw milk contain the exact nutrients, fibers, and enzymes that are required to digest and metabolize their natural sugars.

For instance, the minerals required to digest sugar are calcium, phosphorous, chromium, magnesium, cobalt, copper, zinc and manganese. Sugar cane in its natural form is rich in these vitamins and minerals. It also contains vitamins A, C, B1, B2, B6, niacin, iron, and pantothenic acid, which work synergistically with natural sugar cane's fiber and enzymes to nourish the body. The natural fibers specific to the sugar cane help slow down the absorption of the sugars and prevent the sharp rise in blood sugar levels associated with refined sugar.

By contrast, refined sugar is devoid of the nutrients and built-in enzyme systems that exist in naturally sweet foods. When we eat refined sugar, the body knows that in order to properly digest the sugar, it needs these minerals and the corresponding enzymes. When these are not eaten along with the sugar, the body tries to adapt by pulling stored nutrients from its own bones and tissues.

For example, when refined sugar is ingested in the absence of the calcium necessary to digest it, calcium is drawn out of the bones and tissues where it is stored. The depletion of calcium from the bones and tissues on a regular—even daily—basis weakens bones, potentially leading to osteoporosis and other degenerative diseases. Doctors often recommend calcium supplements to prevent this depletion; however, if body chemistry is not properly balanced, extra calcium in the body can be toxic.

White flour has an even worse effect on the body. It is, literally, nutritionally deadly and slowly kills you. If you tried to live on white bread alone for 60 days, you would die of malnutrition. The reason is that it lacks the healthy elements found in the whole wheat kernel. In addition to certain B-vitamins (niacin, riboflavin and thiamine), a whole wheat kernel contains two important fibers—bran and germ—necessary for its digestion. These health-giving fibers and nutrients are stripped away from the whole wheat kernel during the refinement and bleaching process that make white flour, leading to a product that is so nutritionally depleted that manufacturers are required by federal law to add certain vitamins back in. That's why we see the word "enriched" on our food labels.

The refining process removes nearly 100 vitamins from the whole wheat kernel, replacing them with synthetic, minute quantities of iron, calcium, B vitamins and vitamin D. Enriched flour is enriched just enough to make sure it doesn't kill you too quickly with the obvious nutritional deficiencies that promote chronic disease and illness.

Because those 100 vitamins, along with the fiber, are missing from white flour products, the body turns to its own bones and tissues in an effort to access the stored nutrients required for digestion of wheat. White flour earns one of the top positions on my list of foods that cause nutrient deficiencies leading to upset body chemistry and resulting in degenerative diseases and obesity.

Refined flour and refined sugar are substances that were never meant to be in the body. For this reason, you will not find them in any of my recipes.

The Six Most Important Foods
for Weight Loss and Good Health

My recipes contain some of the most health-promoting foods you can find. Subsequently, they fit into any eating plan designed to manage weight or to improve a health condition. In addition to adding fresh fruits and vegetables to my diet, along with the elimination of refined white flours and sugars, I have identified six of the most important foods that have helped me lose weight and keep it off. Many of my recipes use one or more of these foods to make delicious and satisfying meals. Here I share with you much of what I have learned about these foods and why they must be an integral part of any weight loss process.

1. COCONUT OIL

Yes, that's right. While Americans have long shunned coconut oil, misled into believing that it's a harmful saturated fat responsible for high cholesterol, obesity, and heart disease, the populations of other countries thrive on a daily dose of its health-promoting properties. In the Polynesian islands, where coconut may comprise up to 60% of the diet, obesity is rare, as is heart disease. After years of quiet research, scientists have shown that coconut oil is the healthiest fat you can eat, dispelling decades of inaccurate information.

While it's true that coconut oil is a saturated fat, it is that very fat and its unique molecular structure that promotes weight loss and provides many other healthful benefits. First of all, it is entirely different from the animal saturated fats. It contains a high amount of lauric acid, the

27

main component found in mother's milk, which is responsible for strengthening the immune system and protecting against viral and bacterial infections. Studies show it has many healing properties, including its effectiveness with treating HIV, SARS, and Crohn's Disease. It has also been shown to prevent cancer, osteoporosis, and diabetes.

The ability of coconut oil to promote weight loss is miraculous. It is considered the only "low fat" fat. All other fats contain 9 calories per gram, whereas coconut oil contains only 6.8 calories per gram. The reason for this is its molecular structure. Most fats are made up of long chains of molecules that get stored in the body to be converted to energy later. Coconut is a medium-chain fat, which means that its molecules are smaller than most other fats. Because it's a medium-chain fat, coconut acts more like a carbohydrate in that it gets burned for energy right away and does not easily store in the body as fat. This in effect increases metabolism and provides a special burst of energy. Because of its ability to speed up metabolism, coconut oil is my oil of choice for weight loss, and should be your choice if you suffer from hypothyroidism (low levels of thyroid hormone).

Most of my recipes call for coconut oil for sautéing, stir-frying, and baking because of its remarkable stability and resistance to oxidation. The molecular structures of most oils break down and lose their healthful qualities when heated. In fact, when oils are heated and used for frying, they become rancid and introduce harmful free radicals into the body when eaten. Coconut oil is the amazing exception, once again due to its medium-chain structure. It has a very high temperature threshold, which makes it an excellent oil for cooking. It can take heat up to about 350 degrees without breaking down the way other fats do. I use it exclusively for any type of pan-frying because it isn't absorbed into fried food like other vegetable oils, so it doesn't contribute extra calories to fried food. It also browns foods beautifully!

You might think that using coconut oil will make all of your food taste like coconuts. On the contrary, the coconut flavor you are most familiar with is an artificial flavor that is sweetened with refined sugar. Coconut oil tastes somewhat buttery and is extremely satisfying. The best way to incorporate coconut into your diet is to use the oil for cooking, the coconut milk for smoothies, soups, dressings and sauces, and sprinkle dried coconut on cereals and yogurt.

What to look for in the store:

Coconut Oil – You should only buy **unrefined, extra virgin, expeller-pressed coconut oil**. It is sold in a clear glass jar or plastic tub. It should be a solid, white in color, with a light texture and a mild taste with a scent of fresh coconut. It is typically sold in a natural foods store.

Coconut Milk – Look for canned coconut milk that does not contain extra ingredients such as carrageenan. You may see dried powdered coconut milk in the store; just pass it by. It's a low quality product in which the fat has been oxidized to some degree.

Unsweetened Dried Coconut (flakes or shredded) – Look for organic, unsweetened dried coconut. You most likely will not find this in a conventional supermarket. Beware of dried coconut that has additives and preservatives such as sulfur dioxide, sulfites, propylene glycol, and of course sugar and sweeteners. I prefer the flakes, but shredded coconut works just as well.

2. STEVIA (pronounced steh vee uh)

One evening in 1997, a friend introduced me to stevia, a completely safe, all natural herbal sweetener. It was just in time, as reports were coming out about the ill effects of Aspartame, the most popular artificial chemical-based sweetener on the market at the time. I had been sugar-free for five years, but I would be lying if I said I wasn't always looking for a way to satisfy my taste for sweet without compromising my health and my weight. Could it be true, an all-natural sweetener with no calories? More than that, it has no effect on blood sugar levels, so it's safe for diabetics? It can withstand high heat so it can be used for cooking and baking, and is 200 to 300 times sweeter than sugar so you don't need a lot of it? If such a sweetener did exist, why hadn't I heard of it, especially since such companies as Coca Cola and Beatrice Foods were already using it in their sugar-free products being sold in other countries?

I discovered that it *is* true, and I've been using stevia in my diet ever since. Back in 1997, it was a relatively new phenomenon and a somewhat obscure product, but today stevia has become one of the most popular and widely used sweeteners in the world. I use stevia almost exclusively in my recipes either as the primary sweetener or blended with other natural sweeteners such as honey. Stevia has become an integral part of my lifestyle of eating foods in their closest to natural form. The following paragraphs about the history of stevia are included to enlighten you and to hopefully change the way you think about sugar and the artificial sweetener industries that have deluded our nation into poor health.

The History of Stevia

Stevia is derived from a plant in the daisy family that was originally found growing in the rainforests of South America. The leaves of the stevia plant, known as "sweet leaf," have been used for over 1500 years by the Guarani Indians of Paraguay as a healing tonic. They also used it to sweeten bitter herbal teas, including mate, a highly nutritional and stimulating tea. M.S. Bertoni, a South American botanical researcher, discovered it in 1887 and introduced it to Europe in 1899. He described the plant in his notes as "a plant with leaves so sweet that a part of one would sweeten a whole gourd full of mate." From that point on, hundreds of scientific studies have been performed on the sweet leaf, documenting its non-toxicity and healthful benefits. The scientific research shows that the leaves of the stevia plant contain many nutrients, including chromium, calcium, magnesium, potassium, iron, beta-carotene, Vitamin C, niacin, and protein. They contain several other compounds called glycosides, which are responsible for the intensely sweet taste, but do not provide calories. The main glycoside in stevia is called stevioside. Research has shown that the body does not digest or metabolize glycosides; therefore, they are not converted to glucose. This important property makes them an ideal sweetening agent for diabetics, hypoglycemics, and those who wish to limit their sugar intake.

Dr. Bertoni wrote articles on the stevia plant in 1905 and 1918, citing its advantages over saccharine, the reigning artificial sweetener of the day. He pointed out that stevia could be employed in its natural state (as pulverized leaves) and it is much cheaper than chemically manufactured saccharine. From Dr. Bertoni's observations, one could conclude that stevia had the potential to economically cripple the sugar and saccharine industries and, therefore, was never aggressively studied or marketed in the United States. Other countries, including Japan, Brazil, China, and South Korea, took notice. Researchers found the stevia plant interesting, resulting in numerous well-designed studies of its safety, chemistry, and stability. The governments of these countries, among others, approved the use of stevia in food products over 30 years ago. Food manufacturers in these countries use stevia extracts to sweeten everything from soy sauce and pickles to Diet Coke. Currently, stevioside holds 52% of the commercial sweetener market in Japan and has become the sweetener of choice in China and throughout the Orient.

U.S. FDA Blocks the Use of Stevia

You won't find stevia being used in food products in the United States. In fact, it is illegal for any manufacturer to advertise it for what it is—a sweetener. The reason for this is economic. Up until the mid-1980's, only a handful of herb companies in the U.S. grew and sold stevia. Very few people knew about it, and only a few health food stores carried it. In 1987, Food and Drug Administration (FDA) inspectors visited herb companies that were growing and selling stevia, telling them to stop using it because it is an "unapproved, unsafe food additive." It is reported that an FDA inspector told a company president they were trying to get people to stop using stevia "because NutraSweet complained to FDA."

Artificial sweeteners like saccharin (Sweet 'n Low), aspartame (NutraSweet & Equal), and sucralose (Splenda) are a big business in this country, as well as sweeteners like sugar, high fructose corn syrup, sorbitol, and maltitol. The manufacturers of these products do not want competition from a natural, inexpensive herb. Since stevia is not a synthetic creation of a pharmaceutical company, it cannot be patented; therefore, anyone is free to market it and profit from it.

In May 1991, the FDA waged an attack against stevia by imposing an alert to block it from being imported into the United States and labeling it an "unsafe food additive." The FDA formally warned the few companies that were selling it to stop using the "illegal herb." In a sinister move, the FDA imposed the same regulations on stevia that they use for new food chemicals, and went so far as to egregiously demand far more extensive studies for stevia than are required for such chemical artificial sweeteners as Sweet 'n Low, Nutrasweet, and Splenda.

During this time, the American Herbal Products Association (AHPA) was working to convince the FDA of the safety of stevia. Doug Kinghorn, Ph.D., one of the world's leading authorities on stevia and other non-nutritive sweeteners, conducted a professional review of the studies and literature on stevia. His report concluded that

33

there was nothing in the research, either historically or currently, to indicate that stevia has any ill effects on human health (the same cannot be said of saccharine, aspartame, or sucralose). The AHPA petitioned the FDA to have stevia officially placed on the GRAS (Generally Regarded as Safe) list, supported by vast historical records on stevia, studies by interested researchers in other countries, and references to numerous toxicological studies conducted during the approval process in Japan. The petition pointed out that stevia should be exempted from food additive regulations, since it is a food, which has already been recognized as safe due to its long history of food use. Foods with a long history of safe use are exempted by law from the extensive laboratory tests required of new food chemicals. Despite the mountain of evidence of stevia's safety, the FDA rejected the petition. Soon thereafter, stevia disappeared from the shelves of the few health food stores where it had been sold.

Stevia's Sweet Return

In 1993, the FDA attempted to limit the availability of dietary supplements and herbal products. To the FDA's surprise, there was a huge public outcry against what was seen as an intrusion on a person's right to self-medicate using herbs and supplements. A band of senators, members of Congress and several natural foods companies sided with the public and a law was enacted in 1994, which prevented the FDA from placing restrictions on dietary supplements. The Dietary Supplement Health and Education Act essentially lifted the import ban and opened the door for stevia's return to the United States—not as a sweetener, however, but as a dietary supplement. According to the FDA, stevia's natural sweetness is a "technical effect" that cannot be used for marketing purposes. And because the FDA has not removed the supposed "unsafe food additive" label from stevia, the mainstream and natural foods industries will not use it in their products as a sweetener or dietary supplement. An exception to this is some brands of whey protein powders, which blatantly boast the inclusion of stevia as the sweetening agent instead of other harmful artificial sweeteners often found in similar products. The original homemade version of Dee's Mighty Muffins™ (see index) contains stevia, but I was hard pressed to find a commercial bakery that would use it!

Stevia's Health Benefits

In addition to its natural sweetening qualities, stevia has many health benefits. There have been over 500 scientific studies performed on stevia since it was first discovered in 1899. The results of the studies reveal that stevia has the following positive effects on human health when added to the daily diet:

- Stevia is effective in regulating and normalizing blood sugar levels in people who suffer from diabetes and hypoglycemia.
- Stevia aids the weight loss process because it contains no calories and may, therefore, be used in recipes that satisfy the sweet tooth and balance the diet, eliminating feelings of deprivation or lack of variety. A small amount of stevia goes a long way and will help to reduce cravings for sweets and fatty foods.
- Stevia inhibits the growth of oral bacteria. This may explain why regular users of mouthwashes and toothpastes containing stevia are less susceptible to

colds and flu. Studies also show improvement with bleeding gum problems.

- Stevia can be applied externally to the skin to rapidly heal wounds and cuts, and to clear up eczema, dermatitis, and acne.
- Stevia contains inulin, a natural fiber that stimulates the growth of helpful intestinal bifidobacteria. This may explain why stevia improves digestion and soothes an upset stomach.

What to look for in the store:

You will find stevia in the nutrition section of natural food stores along side the vitamins, herbs, and dietary supplements. Some natural food stores have gotten brave and place them next to other natural sweeteners such as honey and syrups. Some major grocery chains now carry it in their natural foods sections.

Liquid Stevia Extract – This is my favorite because it blends easily into recipes and mixes into cold drinks. It is usually sold in 1 ounce, 2 ounce, or 4 ounce amber colored bottles with a medicine dropper screw cap. It's a clear liquid with a water, glycerin, alcohol, or grapefruit seed extract base. Its taste is extremely sweet, so carefully add it to recipes as not to over-sweeten. If you use too much, you may be turned off to its taste for good. Most natural food stores have their own store brand product of liquid stevia.

Bulk Stevia Powder and Stevia Packets –
This is a white powdered extract blended with a
filler, usually fructooligosaccharides—FOS, a
plant based fiber. Bulk stevia powder comes in
a small plastic bottle with a cap. It is just as
sweet as the clear liquid extracts. Powdered
stevia is also sold in green colored packets
(similar to the pink, blue, and yellow packets).
The powder in the packets is not as sweet as the
liquid or bulk powder and it doesn't dissolve
well into cold drinks. The bulk stevia powder
or stevia from packets can be used in recipes
instead of liquid, but you'll have to use a little
more of it. I am not a fan of the powders,
mainly because of the fillers that are used.
Beware of powdered stevia that contains
maltodextrin, a food additive derived from
cornstarch that may contain MSG.

Dark Stevia Concentrate – This is also a
liquid form of stevia that comes in the same
type of amber bottle; however, the extract is a
dark liquid and has a licorice taste. It makes a
good substitute for brown sugar and molasses
because, when blended with other foods, it
turns them dark in color.

Whole Leaf Stevia – This is the real deal. The
whole dried stevia leaves are crumbled or
crushed into a green powder. These are usually
found in the bulk herb section of natural food
stores or herb stores. The leaves can be added

to teas or soups. You can also make your own liquid extract.

Using Stevia in Place of Sugar

It is nearly impossible to give an exact measurement for replacing sugar in recipes due to the intense sweetness of stevia. There are also a few other drawbacks. We only need minute amounts of stevia; therefore, it doesn't add the type of volume to a recipe that a cup of sugar does. Baked goods will not rise the way those that are baked with sugar will. Sugar is a catalyst for the fermentation process of yeast and helps retain moisture in baked goods. Stevia does not have the same effect. I have had to experiment with the amount of stevia I use in my recipes, and you will have to do the same. My recommendation is that you start with a small amount until you become familiar with its taste, and add more if you want more sweetness. DO NOT USE TOO MUCH STEVIA. Too much stevia will result in a noticeable aftertaste, and you may be turned off to it forever.

Here are some approximate measurements for using stevia in place of sugar:

1 teaspoon Stevia Liquid...............................1 cup sugar

1½ to 2 tablespoons white Stevia powder, bulk...... 1 cup sugar

18 to 24 individual Stevia packets......................1 cup sugar

2 teaspoons dark Stevia concentent..............1 cup brown sugar

3. OMEGA-3 FATS: FLAXSEED OIL and FLAX SEEDS

Most American diets are deficient in omega-3 fats. That is unfortunate since our bodies need these fats for proper protection of our cell membranes and to help metabolize other fats in our diet. Like the fat contained in coconut oil, omega-3 fats raise your metabolism and lower your triglyceride levels. They also help your body burn fat more efficiently. Omega-3s are found in flax seeds and flax seed oil, borage seeds and borage seed oil, hemp oil, fish oil, cold-water fish such as tuna, salmon and sardines, walnuts, and leafy greens. You can also buy eggs containing omega-3 fatty acids. Flaxseed oil, sometimes called just flax oil, is one of the most efficient ways to get omega-3's into your body. It is easily absorbed when eaten with other foods. You will find many of these foods sprinkled throughout my recipes as a way of incorporating omega-3 fats into your diet.

Flaxseed Oil

Ann Louise Gittleman, Ph.D., considered the First Lady of Nutrition in the United States, claims "any dietary or weight loss program undertaken without the addition of the essential nutrients in flaxseed oil is destined to fail." When changing the way you eat in order to lose weight, flaxseed oil helps tremendously. It has an amazing ability to provide satiety. You will feel full for a sustained period of time after adding one tablespoon of oil at a meal because the omega-3 fats cause the stomach to retain food for a longer period of time as compared to fat-free or low fat foods. In my recipes, I blend it into yogurt, smoothies, salad dressings, and pure maple syrup.

Flaxseed oil is very sensitive to light and heat; therefore, *it should never be heated or used for cooking.* The label should read that it is expeller pressed, indicating that the oil was not exposed to heat during the pressing process. If exposed to heat and light for extended periods of time, flax oil loses all of its nutritional and beneficial qualities because it will turn rancid.

Whole Flax Seeds

These are the seeds that the oil is pressed from. The seeds in their whole or ground form provide the same health benefits as the oil along with added fiber. Flax seeds are small, reddish-brown, or golden yellow seeds slightly larger in size than sesame seeds. The oil in whole flaxseeds is bound tightly within the seed and can therefore withstand the heat of baking, which makes them ideal for adding to baked goods and meatloaves. They add nutrition and fiber when added to recipes.

Ground Flax Seeds (also called flax meal)

Whole flaxseeds can be ground to a fine granular consistency in a coffee grinder. Flax seeds should be used soon after grinding, as exposure to air and light oxidizes the oil more rapidly. When adding flaxseeds to a recipe, it is best to use them in the ground form because they are easier to digest. Ground flax seed can stand in for all of the oil or shortening called for in a recipe because of its high oil content. If a recipe calls for 1/3 cup of oil, use 1 cup of ground flax seed to replace the oil — a 3:1 substitution ratio. When flax seed is used instead of oil, baked goods tend to brown more rapidly.

What to look for in the store:

Flaxseed Oil - Purchase flaxseed oil in the refrigerated case of the nutrition section of your natural foods store. Some major grocery chains now carry it in their natural foods sections. It should be contained in a dark bottle, sealed tightly, and kept refrigerated at all times. The bottle should list an expiration date of no longer than four months from the date of pressing to ensure freshness and nutritional potency. To extend freshness, you may freeze unopened bottles of flaxseed oil and thaw them in the refrigerator prior to use. Always keep flaxseed oil refrigerated. Do not buy flaxseed oil that is on the store shelf at room temperature in a glass or plastic bottle. Flaxseed oil kept at room temperature is not of high quality and may possibly go rancid.

Flaxseed Oil Gel Caps - Flaxseed oil may also be purchased in gel caps. Flaxseed oil in gel cap form may be kept at room temperature, which makes them ideal for when you are traveling. The downfall with taking gel caps is that you need to take six of them to provide the same amount of omega-3s in one tablespoon of oil. Also, using oil in it's pure form is better absorbed by the body due to the fact that you don't have to digest the gel caps before your body can use the oil. Only use gel caps when you are traveling and cannot keep fresh flaxseed oil handy.

I recommend purchasing a brand of flax oil that is organic and contains lignans. Lignans are particles of ground flax seeds that exhibit strong antioxidant properties.

Whole Flax Seeds – Most natural food stores carry whole flax seeds in the bulk food sections. Organic flax seeds are preferable.

Ground Flax Seeds (also called flax meal) – These come in sealed foil packaging to preserve freshness.

4. OAT BRAN

Oat bran is the edible, outermost layer of the whole oat kernel. I chose it as the main ingredient in my flourless muffins for its many health benefits. Oat bran is a whole grain that contains protein, healthy fat, minerals, and the B complex vitamins—niacin, thiamin, and riboflavin. Oat bran's most virtuous and versatile component is its soluble fiber. Like stevia, it is recognized as a food and an herb. Unlike stevia, the FDA *loves* oat bran. In January 1997, the FDA passed a unique ruling that allowed oat bran to be registered as the first cholesterol-reducing food, for its ability to bind to blood cholesterol and effectively flush it from the body.

Because oat bran is high in fiber, it promotes weight loss by reducing cravings, stabilizing blood sugar levels,

42

and by providing a prolonged feeling of fullness along with a steady boost of energy. It is considered an excellent food for diabetics because the fiber causes dietary sugar to be absorbed more gradually and increases tissue sensitivity to insulin. In fact, studies show that people with type 1 diabetes who incorporate oat bran into their balanced diets reduce their insulin requirements.

The fiber in oat bran helps regulate bowel function and can alleviate constipation—a health problem that many overweight people suffer from which can lead to a number of bowel diseases, including colon cancer. The soluble fiber in oat bran activates white blood cells, which in effect strengthens the immune system and may prevent some cancers.

Oat bran can be eaten raw or cooked. Prepared as a hot cereal like oatmeal, it serves as a nice breakfast food. I also use it in place of breadcrumbs in recipes. And of course, you can make muffins with it.

What to look for in the store:

Raw Oat Bran – Most natural food stores carry raw oat bran in the bulk food section. I recommend buying it in bulk.

5. FLOURLESS BREAD (SPROUTED WHOLE GRAIN BREAD)

This is another one of those "too good to be true" foods. Giving up flour and sugar doesn't mean giving up bread. In fact, when you give up eating refined white bread you're not giving up anything at all, because there isn't any nutrition in it. There is a process, called sprouting, which releases the vital nutrients stored in whole grains and makes delicious breads that are richer in protein and vitamins than breads baked from dry grains ground into flour. The bread contains significantly higher concentrations of calcium, iron, potassium, magnesium, and vitamins A, C, and the B complex vitamins—niacin, thiamin, and riboflavin. The sprouting process causes a natural change that makes the protein and carbohydrates in the grains easier for the body to digest and use. The baking process preserves the nutrients and retains the natural fiber and bran found in the whole grains.

Most of the flourless breads available are made with a combination of organic sprouted grains. These breads are ideal for weight loss because they are filling, regulate blood sugar levels, and do not cause cravings. Believe me, you will not want to overeat on this bread! I use it for sandwiches, French toast, and an amazingly delicious stuffing mix.

What to look for in the store:

Flourless Breads and Bread Products – You will find flourless breads in the natural food store and in some major grocery chains. They are highly perishable due to their lack of chemical preservatives and are usually kept in the freezer or refrigerated section.

There are several companies that make their own brand of flourless breads. My favorite brand of flourless bread is called Ezekiel 4:9, made by a company called Food For Life. They have five varieties of sliced bread: Sprouted Wheat, Low-Sodium Sprouted Wheat, 7-Grains, Cinnamon Raisin, and Sesame. They also make burger buns, hot dog buns, tortillas, bagels, and English muffins. For those who want to go flourless, it's the greatest thing since, well, sliced bread!

6. APPLE CIDER VINEGAR

Raw, unfiltered, organic apple cider vinegar is different from refined and distilled vinegars found in most grocery stores. The best apple cider vinegar comes from pressed apples matured in wooden barrels. Natural apple cider vinegar is the same cloudy, light-brownish color as natural apple juice. When held up to the light, you should see floating particles of a cobweb like substance that is called the "mother."

This amazing Mother of Vinegar is naturally formed from the pectin and apple residues and appears as strand-like chains of connected protein molecules. The more raw and unfiltered the cider vinegar, the more "mother" shows in the bottle. Any vinegar that is clear and has no "mother" has no nutritional value.

Apple cider vinegar has been highly regarded throughout history. The venerated Greek healer, Hippocrates, used apple cider vinegar for its many healing and cleansing properties. Apple cider vinegar is made from pressing fresh apples; therefore, it is not surprising that the vinegar contains as many health benefits as the apple itself. Apples are one of the richest sources of potassium, an important mineral for keeping the arteries of the body soft, flexible, and resilient, and for fighting off bacteria and viruses.

Among it many health benefits, apple cider vinegar has been proven to help in reducing weight. In the early 1950's, D.C. Jarvis, a Vermont country doctor, published a book describing how he used apple cider vinegar to successfully treat a number of common ailments as well as chronic conditions such as high blood pressure, arthritis, and overweight.

Dr. Jarvis proved that adding apple cider vinegar to the daily diet leads to gradual weight loss. There is good science behind why this is true. Apples are a good source of pectin—a soluble fiber similar to the fiber that is in oat bran. Apple cider vinegar contains the same amount of pectin as apples. In addition to improving insulin sensitivity, soluble fiber can help you feel more full and more satisfied, and reduce the number of calories your body will absorb.

Apple cider vinegar is an acid, which assists in the digestion of protein, which in turn is needed for the production of insulin. Insulin is necessary for converting glucose to energy—the energy required to maintain an active, fat-burning metabolism.

The acetic acid in apple cider vinegar improves the absorption of iron from the food we eat. Iron is a necessary nutrient that is responsible for attracting the oxygen that is essential for burning energy in the body. In effect, apple cider vinegar increases energy consumption in the body, thereby making it a supportive food for weight loss.

Incorporating apple cider vinegar into your daily diet is simple. Based on the work of Dr. Jarvis and others, it is recommended to add 1 to 2 teaspoons of apple cider vinegar to a glass of pure water and drink before meals three times per day. Sweeten with stevia if necessary. If it

46

is too difficult to drink apple cider vinegar before each meal, you can drink one in the morning before breakfast, one before retiring at night, and one at another time during the day when it is convenient. I also use apple cider vinegar in salad dressings.

What to look for in the store:

Raw Unfiltered Organic Apple Cider Vinegar – You will find raw apple cider vinegar in natural food stores. It should be dark brown and the "mother" should be clearly visible.

Light Yet Hearty Breakfasts

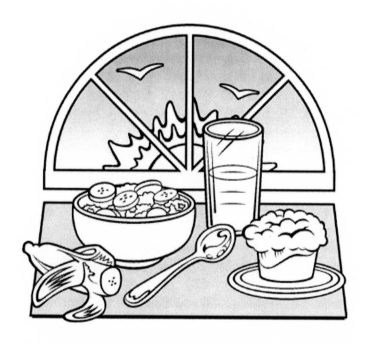

Breakfast is my favorite meal of the day, and it really is the most important meal. Eating in the morning stokes your metabolism and gets your body burning calories early in the day. The best foods to eat for breakfast are high fiber whole grains, low fat proteins, and fruits.

High Protein Fruit Smoothie

This is a refreshingly simple and nutritious breakfast or snack idea and an easy way to incorporate flax oil into your diet.

Makes 1 serving

- 1 cup fresh or frozen fruit (strawberries, blueberries, raspberries, peaches, etc,) or a whole banana
- 1 scoop whey protein powder, vanilla flavored (stevia sweetened only)
- 1 cup almond milk, unsweetened
- ½ cup water
- 1 tablespoon flaxseed oil
- 2-3 drops liquid stevia extract, or to taste

Place all ingredients in a blender. Blend until rich and creamy, approximately 2-3 minutes. Drink immediately.

Nutrition per serving: 209 calories; 15 g Total Fat; 1 g saturated fat; 7 g protein; 12 g carbohydrates; <1 g dietary fiber; 0 mg cholesterol; 127 mg sodium.

Carob Peanut Butter Smoothie

This one is loaded with the good fats, good protein and natural fiber.

Makes 1 serving

- 1 cup almond milk, unsweetened
- ½ banana, frozen
- 1 scoop whey protein powder, vanilla flavored (stevia sweetened only)
- 1 tablespoon natural peanut butter
- 1 teaspoon unsweetened carob powder
- 1 tablespoon flax seed oil
- 1 tablespoon ground flax seeds (also called flax meal)
- 2-3 drops liquid stevia extract, or to taste

Place all ingredients in a blender. Blend until rich and creamy, approximately 2-3 minutes. Drink immediately.

Nutrition per serving: 456 calories; 27 g Total Fat; 2 g saturated fat; 31 g protein; 21 g carbohydrates; 3 g dietary fiber; 0 mg cholesterol; 355 mg sodium.

Dee's Favorite Breakfast

This really is my favorite breakfast! I eat it nearly every day!

Makes 1 serving

- 1 cup plain non-fat yogurt, preferably organic
- ½ teaspoon cinnamon
- 3 drops liquid stevia extract to taste
- 2 tablespoons ground flax seeds (also called flax meal)
- 2 tablespoons raw wheat germ or raw oat bran
- 1 tablespoon flax oil
- 1 tablespoons unsweetened shredded coconut or coconut flakes (preferably organic and unsulfured)
- 1 tablespoon sliced raw almonds
- 1 cup sliced fruit

Combine yogurt, cinnamon, and stevia. Stir to mix. Add flax seeds, wheat germ or oat bran and flax oil. Mix well until all oil is absorbed. Top with coconut, almonds, and fruit. Enjoy! This is a complete breakfast.

Follow breakfast with a cup of jasmine green tea.

Nutrition per serving: 382 calories; 15 g Total Fat; 3 g saturated fat; 17 g protein; 45 g carbohydrates; 8 g dietary fiber; 0 mg cholesterol; 177 mg sodium.

Vegetable Omelet

A super way to get your veggies in the morning!

Makes 1 serving

- 2 omega-3 enriched organic brown eggs
- 1 tablespoon coconut oil
- 1/8 cup coconut milk
- dash of Herbamare
- dash of black pepper
- 2 cloves garlic, minced
- ¼ cup chopped green onion
- 1 cup chopped vegetables including mushrooms, tomatoes, bell pepper, zucchini, and fresh spinach.

Crack eggs into a bowl and add a small amount of milk and a dash of sea salt and black pepper. Blend with a wire whisk and set aside.

In a medium skillet, sauté garlic, peppers and mushrooms in coconut oil over medium heat until peppers are tender. Add eggs, spinach and green onion and cook until done. Serve immediately with salsa if desired.

Variations: You may add fresh herbs such as basil, parsley, cilantro and thyme, and you can add chicken or other poultry.

Nutrition per serving: 386 calories; 30 g Total Fat; 19 g saturated fat; 17 g protein; 14 g carbohydrates; 2 g dietary fiber; 425 mg cholesterol; 173 mg sodium

Spinach and Salmon Frittata

A great way to add Omega-3's to your Morning!

Makes 6 servings (serving = 1/6 of pan)

- 2 tablespoons coconut oil
- 1 bunch green onions, trimmed and chopped
- 3 ounces goat cheese
- 8 eggs (omega-3 enriched)
- ¼ teaspoon black pepper
- 4 ounces cooked salmon
- 1 pound fresh baby spinach, chopped

Move oven rack to 4 inches from broiler element. Heat the broiler to high.

Place coconut oil in a wide oven safe skillet. Add onions and cook over medium heat, stirring occasionally, until they become golden.

Meanwhile, beat goat cheese with 1 egg until smooth. Beat in remaining eggs and pepper. Add the chopped spinach to the egg mixture. Cut the salmon into 1 or 2 inch pieces and stir it into the eggs.

When onions are cooked, pour in the eggs and cook over medium heat for 2 minutes. Use a rubber spatula to go around the edges of the pan, allowing fluid egg to flow to the edges. Cover and cook 4 minutes more.

Remove the lid, place the pan under the broiler and cook 30 to 60 seconds, until browned in spots. If the egg is just barely set in the middle, that's good.

Nutrition per serving: 290 calories; 21 g Total Fat; 10 g saturated fat; 22 g protein; 4 g carbohydrates; <1 g dietary fiber; 424 mg cholesterol; 236 mg sodium

100 % Whole Wheat Pancakes or Waffles

Top pancakes or waffles with unsweetened applesauce, 100% fruit spread, vanilla yogurt, fresh fruit, pure maple syrup or brown rice syrup. Avoid imitation syrups and sugar-free syrups.

Makes 16 four-inch pancakes (serving = ˋ1 pancake)

- 2 cups 100% stone ground whole wheat flour
- 2 teaspoons aluminum-free baking powder
- 1 teaspoon baking soda
- ½ teaspoon sea salt
- 2 cups almond milk
- 1 egg, whisked
- ¼ cup unsweetened applesauce

In a medium mixing bowl, combine flour, baking powder, baking soda, and salt. In a separate bowl, whisk the egg, milk and applesauce together. Add to the flour mixture and mix well to make batter.

Heat a griddle or large nonstick skillet over medium heat until hot. Pour batter on griddle ¼ cup at a time, making sure the edges of each pancake don't touch. Cook until golden brown and bubbles appear on top of the pancakes. Flip and continue cooking until the other side is golden brown.

To make waffles: Prepare batter as above. Preheat waffle iron until ready for cooking. Pour batter onto hot waffle iron and cook until golden brown. Blueberry pancakes: add 1-cup fresh or frozen blueberries to the batter. Banana-Nut pancakes: add 1 mashed ripe banana instead of the applesauce and ½ cup chopped walnuts.

Nutrition per serving: 62 calories; <1 g Total Fat; 0 g saturated fat; 3 g protein; 11 g carbohydrates; 2 g dietary fiber; 19 mg cholesterol; 170 mg sodium

Ezekiel French Toast

High in fiber, protein, and good oils—sans the powdered sugar—this French Toast quells the desire to cheat!

Makes 1 serving

- 2 slices Ezekiel Bread or other flourless sprouted grain bread
- 2 egg, organic omega-3 enriched
- 1/8 cup coconut milk
- 2 teaspoons cinnamon
- 1 tablespoon pure maple syrup or brown rice syrup
- 1 tablespoon flax oil

Crack eggs into a medium bowl and beat with a wire whisk. Add coconut milk and cinnamon. Whisk again to mix.

Cut slices of bread in half, making 4 halves. Place the bread in the egg mixture and let it soak until it is saturated, about 2 minutes.

Heat coconut oil in a skillet or a griddle over medium heat. Place pieces of egg soaked bread in the skillet. Pour remaining egg mixture over the bread. Cook until golden, then flip and cook until the other side is golden and the egg is cooked through. Transfer to a plate.

While French toast is cooking, mix syrup and flax oil in a small bowl and whisk to mix together. Top French toast with the syrup/flax oil mixture.

Serve immediately. *Avoid imitation syrups and sugar-free syrups.*

Nutrition per serving: 564 calories; 31 g Total Fat; 10 g saturated fat; 22 g protein; 52 g carbohydrates; 8 g dietary fiber; 425 mg cholesterol; 296 mg sodium

Sweet "Fried" Potatoes

Sweet potatoes are more delicious and nutritious than white potatoes.

Makes 3 servings (serving = ½ cup)

- 1 large sweet potato
- 2 tablespoons unrefined coconut oil

Slice the sweet potato into thin slices and then cut each slice in half. Heat oil in a skillet over medium heat. Add potato slices and cover in oil. Cover the skillet and let cook 5-10 minutes, turning often. Let the potatoes brown on each side. Potatoes are done when they are tender enough to cut with a fork.

Serve with vegetable omelet.

Nutrition per serving: 149 calories; 9 g Total Fat; 7 g saturated fat; 3 g protein; 16 g carbohydrates; <1 g dietary fiber; 0 mg cholesterol; 9 mg sodium

Creamy Oat Bran Cereal

Oat bran was the first food to be registered by the FDA as a cholesterol-reducing food. The soluble fiber in oat bran not only flushes cholesterol from the body, but it also helps stabilize blood sugar levels, promotes weight loss, and may help prevent some types of cancer.

Makes 2 servings (serving = ¾ cup)

- 2/3 cup raw oat bran
- 2 cups water
- 2 teaspoons cinnamon
- 4-6 drops liquid stevia extract, or to taste
- 2 tablespoons unsweetened dried coconut flakes
- 2 tablespoons almond milk

Place water and oat bran in a saucepan over medium high heat. Bring to a boil while stirring. Reduce heat to low and simmer for 10 minutes until thick and creamy, stirring occasionally. Transfer to bowls.

To each bowl add 2-3 drops stevia extract, 1 teaspoon cinnamon, and almond milk. Stir to mix well. Sprinkle with coconut flakes. Serve immediately.

VARIATION: Try this recipe with oatmeal too! Just replace the oat bran with rolled oats. Whole oats also contain oat bran, so you still get the great benefit of the soluble fiber contained in the bran.

Nutrition per serving: 159 calories; 6 g Total Fat; 3 g saturated fat; 6 g protein; 20 g carbohydrates; 8 g dietary fiber; 0 mg cholesterol; 9 mg sodium

Homemade Granola

This naturally sweet and crunchy granola is great as a snack, sprinkled over yogurt and berries, or in a bowl with cold milk.

Makes 15 cups (serving = ¼ cup)

- 4 cups rolled oats
- 2 cups unsweetened shredded coconut, organic and unsulfured
- 3 cups sliced raw almonds
- ¾ cup coconut oil, liquid at room temperature
- ½ cup raw unfiltered honey
- ½ cup raisins
- 1 ½ cup small dried apricots, diced
- 1 cup small dried figs, diced
- 1 cup dried cherries
- 1 cup dried cranberries
- 1 cup raw cashews

Preheat oven to 350 degrees. Toss the oats, coconut, and almonds together in a large bowl. Whisk together the oil and honey in a small bowl. Pour the oil/honey mixture over the oat mixture and stir with a wooden spoon until completely coated. Pour onto a 13x18 inch baking sheet. Bake, stirring occasionally with a spatula, until the mixture turns a nice, even golden brown, about 45 minutes. Remove granola from the oven and allow to cool, stirring occasionally. Add the apricots, figs, cherries, cranberries, and cashews. Store the cooled granola in an airtight container.

Nutrition per serving: 165 calories; 10 g Total Fat; 5 g saturated fat; 3 g protein; 17 g carbohydrates; 1 g dietary fiber; 0 mg cholesterol; 4 mg sodium

Special thanks to Michelle Trepp, one of my nutrition students, for contributing this recipe.

Awesome
Salads & Dressings

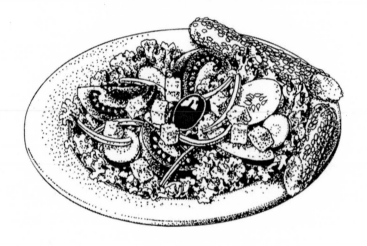

Salads are nature's way of filling us with the life-giving energy contained in vegetables and fruits.

Romaine Salad

A basic salad that contains lettuce, carrots, and celery boosts the immune system.

Makes 2 ½ cups salad, enough for 1 person

- 1 cup sliced romaine lettuce, preferably organic
- 1/2 stalk celery, sliced
- 1 green onion
- 1 grated carrot
- ¼ yellow bell pepper, sliced
- ¼ cup fresh parsley, chopped
- 1 whole red beet, cooked
- ¼ cup Ezekiel Croutons (see index)

Place the romaine in a medium bowl. Add the other vegetables and toss gently. Top with Pepita Cilantro Dressing (see index). Serve immediately.

Nutrition per serving: 140 calories; 3 g Total Fat; 0 g saturated fat; 5 g protein; 24 g carbohydrates; 2 g dietary fiber; 0 mg cholesterol; 230 mg sodium

Rainbow Salad

This one is loaded with color and flavor!

Makes 4 servings (serving = 2 cups)

- 1 head romaine or any fresh organic lettuce, washed and torn
- 1-2 large organic carrots, grated
- 10 black olives
- 1 ripe avocado, sliced
- 1 cup garbanzo beans
- ½ cup walnuts, chopped
- 2 hard boiled organic eggs, chopped
- 3-4 tablespoons chopped fresh basil
- 2 red roasted peppers, sliced
- 1 cup torn red cherry tomatoes
- sliced red onion to taste

Place all ingredients in a large bowl and toss. Top with Sweet Herb Vinaigrette or Creamy Avocado dressing (see index).

Nutrition per serving: 378 calories; 23 g Total Fat; 3 g saturated fat; 13 g protein; 31 g carbohydrates; 4 g dietary fiber; 149 mg cholesterol; 335 mg sodium

Baby Greens Salad

Tender baby greens are easy to put together, especially since you can buy them already washed and bagged!

Makes 4 servings (serving = 2 ½ cups)

- 8 cups organic baby greens or spring mix
- 1 cup diced or shredded red beet, raw
- 1 grated carrot
- 1/2 of a medium size zucchini, sliced
- ½ avocado
- 1 hard boiled egg
- 1 cup tri-colored bell peppers, sliced into thin strips
- ¼ cup toasted pepitas (green pumpkin seeds)
- crumbled feta cheese for garnish

Place the salad greens in a large bowl. Top with the other veggies, arranging into a nice colorful salad. Garnish top of the salad with feta cheese and pepitas. Serve with vinaigrette or avocado dressing.

Nutrition per serving: 225 calories; 12 g Total Fat; 4 g saturated fat; 10 g protein; 20 g carbohydrates; 3 g dietary fiber; 66 mg cholesterol; 332 mg sodium

Two Tone Beet, Spinach and Feta Salad

Beets are a sweet treat that add variety and color to your salads.

Makes 4 servings (serving = 3 cups)

- 3 tablespoons olive oil
- 2 tablespoons apple cider vinegar
- 2 tablespoons Dijon mustard
- ½ teaspoon each: dried tarragon or basil and minced garlic
- ¼ teaspoon each: sea salt and ground black pepper
- 8 cups packed organic baby spinach or spring mix
- 4 medium yellow beets, cooked and sliced
- 4 medium red beets, cooked and sliced
- 1 cup (4 ounces) crumbled feta
- ¼ cup pine nuts

To cook the beets, preheat oven to 400 degrees. Leave about 1 inch stems and tails on beetroot. Scrub beets and place in baking dish with a little water. Cover and bake the beets until tender (25-45 minutes). Cool then peel and quarter.

For the salad dressing, combine oil, vinegar, mustard, tarragon, garlic, and salt and pepper in a jar with a tight fitting lid. Shake well. Dressing may be prepared and refrigerated up to 5 days before serving.

In a large bowl, combine spinach or spring mix and beets. Add the dressing, toss well to coat. Transfer mixture to 4 serving plates; top with cheese and nuts.

Nutrition per serving: 367 calories; 23 g Total Fat; 7 g saturated fat; 12 g protein; 28 g carbohydrates; 3 g dietary fiber; 25 mg cholesterol; 876 mg sodium

Gold Beets with Walnut Vinaigrette

Walnut oil brings a luscious flavor to this salad along with its nutritional advantages. Like the nuts from which it is pressed, walnut oil is rich in omega-3 fatty acids.

Makes 4 servings (serving = ½ cup)

- 1 pound gold beets, trimmed
- 2 teaspoons balsamic vinegar
- 2 teaspoons apple cider vinegar, raw unfiltered organic
- ¼ teaspoon sea salt
- 1 tablespoon toasted walnut oil, organic
- 3 to 4 tablespoons extra virgin olive oil
- 1 tablespoon Italian parsley, chopped
- ¼ teaspoon black pepper
- 1 ounce goat cheese

To cook the beets, preheat oven to 400 degrees. Leave about 1 inch stems and tails on beetroot. Scrub and put in baking dish with a little water. Cover and bake the beets until tender (25-45 minutes). Cool then peel and quarter.

While the beets are baking prepare the vinaigrette. Combine vinegars and salt and add the oils. While the beets are still warm, dress with the vinaigrette and parsley. Add more vinegar to taste. Season with pepper.

Nutrition per serving: 205 calories; 16 g Total Fat; 3 g saturated fat; 4 g protein; 12 g carbohydrates; 1 g dietary fiber; 7 mg cholesterol; 247 mg sodium.

Chilled Bean Medley

This combination of beans and seasonings makes a great salad for picnics and pot lucks. It's great for snacking too!

Makes 16 servings (serving = ½ cup)

- 1 can (15 ounce) organic garbanzo beans
- 1 can (15 ounce) organic white kidney beans
- 1 can (15 ounce) organic red kidney beans
- 1 cup fresh or frozen organic baby lima beans
- 1 can (15 ounce) black eyed peas
- 1 cup fresh or frozen green beans, cooked
- 1 cup chopped scallions
- ½ cup chopped Italian parsley, for garnish
- 1 cup Sweet Herb Vinaigrette (see index)

Drain canned beans, rinse thoroughly with water and drain again. Cook fresh or frozen green beans and lima beans, and then add them to the drained beans.

To assemble salad: Toss beans together in a large bowl. Pour in the vinaigrette, sprinkle on the scallions, and toss again. Cover and refrigerate overnight before serving. Garnish with chopped parsley. Serve at room temperature.

Special thanks to Sue Wiedenhoeft, one of my nutrition students, for contributing this recipe.

Nutrition per serving: 176 calories; 10 g Total Fat; 1 g saturated fat; 6 g protein; 16 g carbohydrates; 1 g dietary fiber; 0 mg cholesterol; 304 mg sodium.

Spicy Cole Slaw

Safflower mayonnaise is preferred over commercially processed mayonnaise, because the safflower oil is expeller pressed and vitamin E, a natural antioxidant, is added to preserve the oil.

Makes 12 servings (serving = 1/2 cup)

Dressing:
- 1 cup lite safflower mayonnaise
- 2 tablespoons toasted sesame oil
- 2 tablespoons mirin
- ¼ cup chili sauce
- 3 tablespoons freshly squeezed lime juice
- 1 tablespoon grated ginger
- 1/8 teaspoon coarse sea salt
- ¼ teaspoon freshly ground pepper
- 2 teaspoons toasted sesame seeds

Slaw:
- ½ small head red cabbage (about 1 pound)
- ½ head napa cabbage (about 1 pound)

- 1 turnip, peeled (about 9 ounces)
- 1 small daikon, peeled (about 8 ounces)
- 1 large carrot, peeled
- 4 scallions, thinly sliced on the diagonal
- 1 red bell pepper, seeded and thinly sliced
- ¼ cup finely chopped fresh mint leaves
- ¼ cup finely chopped fresh cilantro

Dressing: In a medium bowl, whisk together mayonnaise, sesame oil, mirin, chili sauce, lime juice, ginger, salt, pepper, and sesame seeds; set aside.

Slaw: Slice red and napa cabbages very thinly. Place in a large bowl and set aside.

Grate the turnip, daikon and carrot using a box grater or food processor. Add to bowl of cabbage along with scallions, bell pepper, mint and cilantro. Add reserved dressing, and toss to combine. Cover with plastic wrap, and let sit at least 2 hours in the refrigerator, but preferably overnight. Serve chilled. Will keep in the refrigerator for up to 4 days.

Nutrition per serving: 139 calories; 10 g Total Fat; 0 g saturated fat; 2 g protein; 10 g carbohydrates; 1 g dietary fiber; 0 mg cholesterol; 241 mg sodium.

Tasty Tuna Salad

Adding veggies to your tuna salad helps ensure you get adequate amounts of vegetables in your daily diet.

Makes 3 servings (serving = ¾ cup)

- 2 cans (6 ounce) water-packed albacore tuna
- 1 carrot, chopped
- 1 stalk celery, chopped
- ¼ cup walnuts, chopped
- ¼ cup red onion, chopped
- 2 green onions
- 2 tablespoons chopped fresh parsley
- 2 tablespoons lite safflower mayonnaise

In a medium bowl, mix together the tuna, carrot, celery, walnuts, onion, parsley, and mayonnaise. Serve immediately or refrigerate and eat later.

Nutrition per serving: 237 calories; 12 g Total Fat; <1 g saturated fat; 24 g protein; 8 g carbohydrates; 1 g dietary fiber; 0 mg cholesterol; 97 mg sodium.

Omega-3 Egg Salad

The standard American diet is deficient in omega-3 fats. This salad will ensure you get your daily dose!

Makes 1 serving

- 2 hard boiled eggs (omega-3 enriched), cooled, peeled and chopped
- 1/2 carrot, chopped
- 1/2 celery stalk, chopped
- 1 green onion, chopped
- 1 tablespoon chopped walnuts
- 1 teaspoon dried mustard
- 1 tablespoon flaxseed oil
- 1 teaspoon apple cider vinegar
- 1 teaspoon lite safflower mayonnaise
- 1 teaspoon chopped fresh parsley

In a medium bowl, mix together all ingredients. Serve immediately over a leafy green salad or enjoy as a sandwich filling.

Nutrition per serving: 369 calories; 31 g Total Fat; 5 g saturated fat; 15 g protein; 9 g carbohydrates; 1 g dietary fiber; 425 mg cholesterol; 196 mg sodium.

Honey Dijon Dressing

The flavors of honey and Dijon mustard blend nicely in this favorite dressing.

Makes 2 cups (serving = 2 tablespoons)

- 1 cup lite safflower mayonnaise
- ¼ cup Dijon mustard
- ¼ cup extra virgin olive oil
- ¼ cup unfiltered honey
- 1/8 teaspoon onion powder
- 1/8 teaspoon sea salt
- ¾ teaspoon raw unfiltered apple cider vinegar
- 1 garlic clove, minced

Place all ingredients in a blender or mix by hand with a wire whisk until well blended together. Dressing may be kept up to 3 weeks refrigerated.

Nutrition per serving: 95 calories; 7 g Total Fat; 0 g saturated fat; 0 g protein; 6 g carbohydrates; 0 g dietary fiber; 0 mg cholesterol; 170 mg sodium.

Sweet Herb Vinaigrette

This tangy vinaigrette can be used on any salad or as a marinade.

Makes about 1 ½ cups (serving = 1 tablespoon)

- 1 cup extra virgin olive oil
- ½ cup organic unfiltered apple cider vinegar
- 1 teaspoon dried parsley,
- 1 teaspoon dried oregano
- 1 teaspoon dried basil
- 1 teaspoon dried thyme
- 3 cloves fresh garlic, minced
- juice of 1/2 fresh squeezed lemon
- ¼ teaspoon liquid stevia extract
- Herbamare seasoning to taste

Combine all ingredients in a glass jar. Cover the jar, close tightly, and vigorously shake the jar to blend all of the ingredients. Refrigerate. Keeps for up to 3 weeks.

Nutrition per serving: 82 calories; 9 g Total Fat; 1 g saturated fat; 0 g protein; 0 g carbohydrates; 0 g dietary fiber; 0 mg cholesterol; 27 mg sodium.

Creamy Avocado Dressing

A wonderfully creamy and light dressing!

Makes 4 cups (serving = 2 tablespoons)

- 1 can (14 ounce) lite coconut milk
- 3 ripe avocados
- juice from ½ fresh squeezed lime
- 1 cup chopped fresh cilantro
- 4 cloves fresh garlic, minced
- dash cayenne pepper
- 2 tablespoons pepitas, toasted

Place coconut milk in a food processor. Scoop out all of the flesh from the avocadoes and add to the coconut milk. Squeeze the juice from the lime into the coconut milk and avocado mixture. Add the rest of the ingredients and blend until smooth and creamy. Transfer dressing to a jar and refrigerate. Keeps for 3-4 days. If dressing thickens too much, thin it out by adding small amounts of water until the desired consistency is reached.

Nutrition per serving: 50 calories; 4 g Total Fat; 2 g saturated fat; <1 g protein; 2 g carbohydrates; 0 g dietary fiber; 0 mg cholesterol; 14 mg sodium

Pepita Cilantro Dressing

This is the most yummy dressing, very similar to a Mexican Caesar dressing.

Makes 4 cups (serving = 2 tablespoons)

- 1 can (14 ounce) lite coconut milk
- 2 cups water
- ¼ cup cotija cheese
- 1 tablespoon lime juice
- 1 cup parmesan cheese
- 4 cloves garlic
- 1 cup pepitas, toasted
- 1 cup fresh cilantro leaves
- 1 teaspoon raw unfiltered apple cider vinegar
- ¼ cup extra virgin olive oil
- ½ teaspoon sea salt

Place all ingredients into a blender and run until well blended. Store in a tightly sealed container. Dressing keeps for about three days. If dressing thickens too much, thin it out by adding small amounts of water until the desired consistency is reached.

Nutrition per serving: 62 calories; 5 g Total Fat; 2 g saturated fat; 2 g protein; 1 g carbohydrates; 0 g dietary fiber; 3 mg cholesterol; 152 mg sodium

Basil and Pine Nut Pesto

Spoon onto fish, steamed vegetables, or a baked potato.

Makes 2 servings (serving = 1 ½ tablespoons)

- 1 tablespoon toasted pine nuts
- 1 fresh garlic clove
- 2 tablespoons fresh basil
- ½ tablespoon fresh thyme
- 1 tablespoon extra virgin olive oil
- 1 tablespoon flaxseed oil

Place all ingredients into a food processor or blender and puree until well blended.

Nutrition per serving: 147 calories; 16 g Total Fat; 2 g saturated fat; <1 g protein; 2 g carbohydrates; 0 g dietary fiber; 0 mg cholesterol; 3 mg sodium

Sugar-Free Tangy BBQ Sauce

You'll be hard pressed to find a commercially prepared BBQ sauce without sugar. This one is a perfect alternative.

Makes 3 cups (serving size = 2 Tablespoons)

- 2 cups "No Salt Added" Tomato Sauce
- 1 6 ounce can tomato paste, unsalted
- 1 tablespoon blackstrap molasses
- 1 tablespoon Agave nectar
- ½ teaspoon liquid smoke, natural
- 2 tablespoons lemon juice
- ¼ cup chopped onions
- 1 clove of garlic, minced
- 2 tablespoons chili powder
- 2 tablespoons apple cider vinegar, organic raw unfiltered
- 2 tablespoons coconut oil
- 1 tablespoon chopped parsley
- 1 teaspoon dried mustard
- 1 teaspoon smoked paprika
- ¼ teaspoon ground black pepper

Combine all ingredients and simmer 30-45 minutes (or longer) until nice and thick. Add more tomato paste if you need to thicken further.

Nutrition per serving: 32 calories; 1 g Total Fat; 1 g saturated fat; <1 g protein; 4 g carbohydrates; 0 g dietary fiber; 0 mg cholesterol; 13 mg sodium

Meats:
Poultry, Beef, and Fish

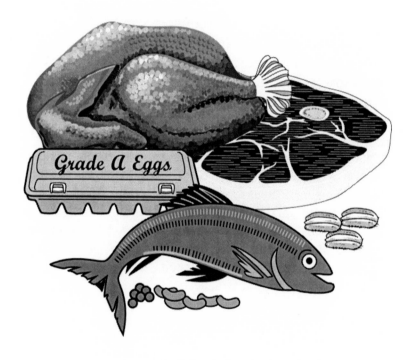

Proteins are the building blocks for muscle development. Protein from animal sources should be lean, and preferably organic.

Sesame Ginger Chicken

Ginger lends a sweet and pungent flavor to the chicken in addition to aiding in digestion.

Makes 6 servings (serving = 4 ounces chicken)

- 1 ½ tablespoon toasted sesame seeds
- 1 tablespoon grated fresh gingerroot
- 3-4 drops liquid stevia extract
- 3 tablespoons reduced sodium wheat free tamari sauce
- 6 boneless, skinless chicken breasts

Combine first four ingredients and set aside. Flatten chicken between 2 sheets of waxed paper to ¼ inch thickness using a meat mallet or rolling pin. Brush half of the soy sauce mixture over chicken, coating both sides. Grill chicken breasts over medium heat 8-10 minutes or until no longer pink (chicken may also be broiled). Frequently baste and turn chicken during cooking and discard any remaining marinade.

Nutrition per serving: 152 calories; 3 g Total Fat; <1 g saturated fat; 29 g protein; <1 g carbohydrates; 0 g dietary fiber; 77 mg cholesterol; 403 mg sodium

Cajun-Spiced Chicken and Rice

Chicken need not be boring!

Makes 4 servings (serving = 4 ounces chicken plus ½ cup rice)

- 1 regular size oven cooking bag
- 1 cup instant brown rice
- 1 green pepper, cubed
- ½ cup chopped onion
- ¼ cup sliced celery
- 2 fresh garlic cloves, minced
- ½ teaspoon thyme leaves
- ¼ teaspoon sea salt
- 1 can (14 ½ ounce) whole tomatoes, cut in half
- ¼ cup water
- 4 to 6 pieces chicken
- ¼ teaspoon cayenne pepper

Preheat oven to 350 degrees. Place cooking bag in 13 x 9 x 2 inch baking pan. Combine rice, green pepper, onion, garlic, celery, thyme and salt in bag. Add tomatoes and water; squeeze bag to blend ingredients. Arrange ingredients in an even layer. Combine cayenne pepper and garlic powder; sprinkle lightly over chicken. Place chicken in bag on top of rice mixture. Close bag with nylon tie; make 6 half-inch slits on top. Bake 1 hour or until tender.

Nutrition per serving: 237 calories; 3 g Total Fat; <1 g saturated fat; 22 g protein; 29 g carbohydrates; 1 g dietary fiber; 51 mg cholesterol; 155 mg sodium

Chicken with Tri-Colored Peppers

The three varieties of bell peppers lend a sweet flavor to chicken.

Makes 4 servings (serving = 4 ounces chicken plus 1 cup peppers and onions)

- 1 regular size oven cooking bag
- ¼ cup water
- 2 teaspoons fresh basil leaves, chopped
- 4 boneless skinless chicken breasts
- sea salt and pepper
- 1 green bell pepper, cut into cubes
- 1 red bell pepper, cut into cubes
- 1 yellow bell pepper, cut into cubes
- 1 medium onion, quartered
- 1 tablespoon butter

Preheat oven to 350 degrees. Place cooking bag in 13 x 9 x 2 inch baking pan. Add water and basil. Squeeze bag to blend ingredients. Rinse chicken; pat dry. Sprinkle chicken with salt and pepper. Place chicken in bag; turn bag to coat with herbed mixture. Place peppers and onion in bag around chicken. Dot chicken and vegetables with butter. Close bag with nylon tie; make 6 half-inch slits in top. Bake 35 minutes or until chicken is tender. Let stand 10 minutes. Spoon peppers and onion over sliced chicken.

Nutrition per serving: 210 calories; 6 g Total Fat; 3 g saturated fat; 29 g protein; 9 g carbohydrates; <1 g dietary fiber; 85 mg cholesterol; 377 mg sodium

Indian Chicken with Eastern Quinoa Pilaf

Coconut milk is a staple food in East Indian cuisine.

Makes 4 servings (serving = 1 cup)

- 1 teaspoon coconut oil
- 1 large onion (for about 1 cup chopped)
- 4 fresh garlic cloves, minced
- 2 teaspoons minced fresh ginger
- 1 pound skinless chicken tenders
- 1 can (14 ounce) lite coconut milk
- ¼ teaspoon ground turmeric
- ¼ teaspoon sea salt
- 1 cup frozen green peas
- 2 cups Eastern Quinoa Pilaf (see index)

Make the Eastern Quinoa pilaf. Heat oil over medium heat in a 12 inch nonstick skillet. Peel and coarsely chop onion, adding it to skillet as you chop. Stir and cook until onion begins to soften, about 2 minutes. Add the garlic and ginger, and stir and cook for 1 minute.

Add chicken to skillet, and raise heat to high. Cook, stirring frequently, until chicken is no longer pink outside, about 3 minutes. Add coconut milk, turmeric and salt, and stir until turmeric is thoroughly mixed in. Bring mixture to a boil. Reduce heat to medium and cook, stirring frequently, until sauce begins to thicken, about 8 minutes.

Meanwhile, measure out the peas and set aside. When the sauce has cooked 6 minutes, stir in the still frozen peas, and continue to cook the final 2 minutes. Serve at once over the Eastern Quinoa pilaf.

Nutrition per serving: 515 calories; 17 g Total Fat; 10 g saturated fat; 40 g protein; 49 g carbohydrates; 4 g dietary fiber; 77 mg cholesterol; 371 mg sodium.

Sesame Chicken and Veggie Stir-Fried Rice

Coconut oil and toasted sesame oil are health promoting and far surpass the quality of any commercially prepared fried rice.

Makes 6 servings (serving = 1 cup)

Chicken:
- 1 lb. boneless, skinless chicken breast, cut into strips or small chunks
- 1 tablespoon reduced sodium soy sauce or wheat-free tamari sauce
- 1 tablespoon toasted sesame oil (expeller pressed, unrefined)
- 4 cloves fresh garlic, minced
- 2 teaspoons fresh ginger, minced
- 1 tablespoon chicken broth or water

Veggies:
- 3 cloves fresh garlic, minced
- 2 teaspoons fresh ginger, minced
- 5 cups mixed vegetables: broccoli, carrots, bell peppers, snow peas, bok choy, cabbage, etc.
- 1 tablespoon coconut oil
- 1 tablespoon toasted sesame oil, (expeller pressed, unrefined)

- 1 teaspoon low sodium soy sauce
- 2 teaspoons toasted sesame seeds
- 1 tablespoon chopped green onions (green parts only)
- 2 eggs, scrambled

Rice:
2 cups Sesame Brown Rice (see index); leave off the garnish for now

Heat a small amount of coconut oil over medium heat in a non-stick skillet. Cook scrambled eggs until done. Remove from heat and set aside.

Place chicken strips in a large bowl. To the chicken strips, add the oil, tamari sauce, garlic, and ginger. Mix thoroughly. In a large frying pan or wok, heat the water or chicken broth over medium heat. Add the chicken mixture and cook until the chicken is done, about 10-15 minutes. Transfer to a bowl and set aside.

In the same large frying pan or wok, heat 1 tablespoon coconut oil over medium heat. Add garlic, ginger, broccoli, and carrots. Cook until broccoli is almost done. Add the rest of the vegetables and the soy sauce and cook until nearly done, about 2 minutes. Add the rice and continue to stir fry until rice is warmed through. Add the scrambled egg. Turn off heat and add bok choy and cabbage at the very end and toss with other vegetables until the cabbage and bok choy are only slightly wilted. Do not overcook bok choy and cabbage. Garnish with green onions and toasted sesame seeds. Serve with cooked chicken.

Nutrition per serving: 317 calories; 13 g Total Fat; 4 g saturated fat; 25 g protein; 23 g carbohydrates; 1 g dietary fiber; 122 mg cholesterol; 357 mg sodium.

Turkey Meatloaf

This is a favorite in my house.

Makes 1 loaf, about 4-6 servings (serving = 5 ounces meatloaf)

- 1 package (1 lb.) lean ground turkey
- 1 cup chopped onion
- 3 cloves garlic, minced
- ½ cup chopped green bell pepper
- 1 tablespoon coconut oil
- 1 large egg
- ½ cup oat bran
- 1 teaspoon dried basil
- 1 teaspoon dried parsley
- 1 teaspoon garlic salt
- ½ teaspoon black pepper
- 1 (8 ounce) can tomato sauce

Heat oven to 350 degrees. In a skillet, heat the oil over medium heat and sauté the onion, bell pepper and garlic until softened, about 5 minutes. Add tomato sauce and spices and cook until it simmers. Remove from heat and set aside.

In a large mixing bowl add the ground turkey, oat bran, egg, and tomato mixture. Mix well with a wooden spoon.

Pack into an 8x4 inch loaf pan. Bake for 50-55 minutes or until no longer pink in center. Let stand at room temperature 5 minutes before slicing.

Nutrition per serving: 238 calories; 11 g Total Fat; 3 g saturated fat; 23 g protein; 13 g carbohydrates; 3 g dietary fiber; 112 mg cholesterol; 209 mg sodium.

Greek Stuffed Turkey Burgers

The flavors of tomatoes and melted feta packed inside the turkey burst in your mouth.

Makes 4 servings (serving = 1 burger)

- 1 pound lean ground turkey
- ½ medium onion, finely diced
- 1 egg
- ½ cup chopped fresh parsley
- ¾ teaspoon dried oregano
- ½ teaspoon cumin
- 4 garlic cloves, minced
- ½ teaspoon sea salt
- ½ teaspoon black pepper
- 1 tomato
- 4 ounces feta cheese
- 1 tablespoon extra virgin olive oil
- parsley sprigs for garnish
- 1 cucumber, sliced

Place ground turkey in a bowl. Add onion and egg and mix with your hands. Add parsley, oregano, cumin, garlic and pepper. Mix, then divide into 5 portions to make burgers.

Slice 4 thin slices of tomato. Cut remainder into wedges or thick slices. Slice feta into 4 thin slices.

Divide each turkey burger in half (a top and a bottom) and flatten each half into a very thin patty. Top 1 half with a slice of tomato and a slice of feta. Place the other half on top and gently seal edges so cheese won't leak out. Repeat with remaining patties.

Brush grill with coconut oil and cook burgers slowly over medium heat until insides are thoroughly cooked, or bake in an oven.

Serve with sliced tomato, parsley sprigs and cucumber slices.

Nutrition per serving: 252 calories; 11 g Total Fat; 2 g saturated fat; 31 g protein; 8 g carbohydrates; <1 g dietary fiber; 145 mg cholesterol; 766 mg sodium.

Turkey Meatballs

Coconut milk again lends its versatile flavor to these savory meatballs.

Makes 4 servings (serving = 4 ounces of meatballs with sauce)

Meatballs:
- 1 pound lean ground turkey
- 2-3 cloves fresh garlic, minced
- 1 teaspoon dried basil
- 1 teaspoon dried parsley
- 1 teaspoon dried oregano
- ¼ teaspoon black pepper
- 2 scallions, chopped (white and green parts)
- 1 egg
- ½ cup oat bran or oatmeal

Sauce:
- 1 pinch dried basil
- 1 pinch dried parsley
- 1 pinch dried oregano
- dash of black pepper
- 1 cup very low sodium chicken broth
- ¼ cup coconut milk

To make meatballs, combine all ingredients into a large bowl and mix together. Form into meatballs and cook in a skillet until done, about 20 minutes.

In a separate saucepan, bring the chicken broth to a simmer. Add the spices and stir. Slowly add coconut milk and stir with a wire whisk. Simmer 5 minutes. Add the sauce to the meatballs and stir. Serve over rice or potatoes.

Nutrition per serving: 256 calories; 12 g Total Fat; 2 g saturated fat; 27 g protein; 10 g carbohydrates; 3 g dietary fiber; 119 mg cholesterol; 123 mg sodium.

Beef and Snow Peas

Snow peas are also known as Chinese snow peas. The French name for this tender legume is mange-tout, *meaning "eat it all."*

Makes 4 servings (serving = 4 ounces beef and 1 cup peas)

- 1 pound beef strip loin (or other lean cut)
- 1 clove garlic, finely chopped
- 1 tablespoon toasted sesame oil (unrefined, expeller pressed)
- sea salt and pepper to taste
- 3 green onions, sliced
- 2/3 cup reduced sodium beef broth
- 1 tablespoon arrowroot
- 2 tablespoons water
- 1 tablespoon reduced sodium wheat free tamari sauce
- 1 teaspoon ground ginger or 2 teaspoons fresh minced ginger root
- 6 ounces snow peas, fresh or frozen (thaw under warm water before cooking)

Remove any fat from beef and cut into 2 inch strips about 1/2 inch thick. Heat a large nonstick skillet or wok over high heat; add the sesame oil. Add the beef and the garlic and stir fry about 3 minutes, stirring constantly. Season with sea salt and pepper. Add the green onions and stir fry about 1 minute.

Stir in broth. Heat to boiling over high heat.

In a small bowl, mix together the water and tamari sauce. Add the arrowroot and mix thoroughly. Add to the beef mixture. Cook, stirring constantly until mixture begins to thicken and boil. Stir in ginger and pea pods and cook uncovered about 2 minutes, stirring constantly. Serve over brown rice.

Nutrition per serving: 258 calories; 13 g Total Fat; 4 g saturated fat; 30 g protein; 6 g carbohydrates; 1 g dietary fiber; 81 mg cholesterol; 523 mg sodium.

Southern Creole

This is another favorite in the McCaffrey household. It's best eaten the following day after all of the vegetables and spices have released their flavors.

Makes 6 servings (serving = 1 turkey sausage, ½ cup rice, and 1 cup veggies)

- 2 tablespoons coconut oil
- 1/3 cup chopped onion
- 4 cloves garlic, minced
- ½ green bell pepper, chopped
- ½ red bell pepper
- 1 can (14 ½ ounce) whole tomatoes, undrained and chopped, preferably organic
- 1 can (15 ounce) tomato sauce, preferably organic
- 1 ½ cups water
- ½ pound fresh okra, sliced or 1 package (10 ounce) frozen sliced okra
- 2 stalks celery with leaves, chopped
- 1 slice lemon
- 2 teaspoons chili powder
- ½ teaspoon sea salt
- ¼ teaspoon black pepper
- ½ teaspoon dried basil
- ½ teaspoon dried thyme
- 2 bay leaves
- 1/8 teaspoon cayenne pepper
- 1 teaspoon fresh parsley, chopped
- 6 links turkey Italian sausage links, cooked and sliced
- 3 cups hot cooked brown rice

Heat oil in a large stockpot over medium heat. Add onion, garlic and bell peppers and sauté until peppers are tender, 2-3 minutes.

Add tomatoes, tomato sauce, water, lemon, celery, okra, chili powder, salt, black pepper, basil, thyme, bay leaf and cayenne. Stir together and mix well. Allow mixture to come to a boil, and then reduce heat to low and cover. Simmer 45 minutes, stirring occasionally.

Stir in shrimp or cooked turkey sausage slices. Cover. Cook 3 minutes or until shrimp turn pink. Remove the lemon slice and bay leaves before serving. Serve over the hot rice and garnish with fresh chopped parsley.

Nutrition per serving: 332 calories; 13 g Total Fat; 6 g saturated fat; 21 g protein; 36 g carbohydrates; 2 g dietary fiber; 70 mg cholesterol; 735 mg sodium.

Bernadette's Cabbage Delight

Cabbage is a cruciferous vegetable that should be a regular part of just about everyone's diet. Cruciferous vegetables are high in fiber, antioxidants, and vitamin K.

Makes 5 servings (serving = 1 cup)

- 1 ½ pound very lean ground beef or ground turkey
- 1 medium onion, chopped.
- 2 cloves garlic, crushed
- ½ head of napa cabbage, coarsely chopped
- 1 can (8 ounce) tomato sauce
- 2 tablespoons lemon juice
- ½ teaspoon pepper
- ½ teaspoon ground nutmeg
- ½ teaspoon ground cinnamon
- 1 teaspoon sea salt

Begin browning the ground beef or turkey in a heavy skillet over high heat. Add the onion and garlic. Cover the pan and let mixture cook for a bit.

Stir cabbage into the beef mixture a little at a time – it will come close to overflowing the skillet. Stir the mixture carefully so it cooks evenly. Re-cover the pan for a few minutes.

When the cabbage starts to wilt, stir in the tomato sauce, lemon juice, pepper, nutmeg, cinnamon, and salt. Cover and let simmer for 5 minutes, then serve.

Special thanks to Bernadette Janas, one of my nutrition students, for contributing this recipe.

Nutrition per serving: 234 calories; 9 g Total Fat; <1 g saturated fat; 28 g protein; 10 g carbohydrates; 2 g dietary fiber; 79 mg cholesterol; 567 mg sodium.

McCaffrey's Yummy Irish Stew

This recipe was developed for a very low sodium diet, which is beneficial for every body!

Makes 12 servings (serving = ½ cup)

- 2 lbs. boneless lamb meat
- 6 medium potatoes
- 3 medium onions, sliced
- 2 carrots, sliced
- ¼ teaspoon black pepper
- ¼ teaspoon dried thyme
- 1 bay leaf
- 2 ½ cups water
- snipped parsley

Cut lamb into 1 inch cubes. Cut potatoes into ½ inch slices. Put lamb, potatoes, carrots and onions into large stew pot. Sprinkle with pepper and thyme and add bay leaf. Add water. Heat to boiling. Reduce heat, cover and simmer until lamb is very tender, 3 to 4 hours.

Before serving, sprinkle with snipped parsley (optional).

Nutrition per serving: 296 calories; 12 g Total Fat; 5 g saturated fat; 17 g protein; 30 g carbohydrates; 1 g dietary fiber; 55 mg cholesterol; 52 mg sodium.

Pan-Grilled Salmon with Pineapple Salsa

Salmon is one of the best sources of omega-3 fatty acids. The best variety is wild caught Alaskan salmon.

Makes 4 servings (serving = 4 ounces salmon and 1/3 cup salsa each)

- 1 cup chopped fresh pineapple
- 2 tablespoons finely chopped red onion
- 2 tablespoons chopped cilantro
- 1 tablespoon rice vinegar
- 1/8 teaspoon ground red pepper
- 1 lb. salmon filets
- 1 tablespoon coconut oil

Combine first 5 ingredients in a bowl; set aside. Heat oil in skillet over medium heat. Cook fish 4 minutes on each side or until it flakes easily when tested with a fork. Top with salsa.

Nutrition per serving: 230 calories; 13 g Total Fat; 4 g saturated fat; 23 g protein; 5 g carbohydrates; 0 g dietary fiber; 74 mg cholesterol; 57 mg sodium.

Steamed Swordfish

This incredibly quick and easy recipe can be used with any fish.

Makes 4 servings (serving = 4-ounce steak)

- 4 (4 ounce) swordfish steaks
- ½ cup lemon juice
- ½ teaspoon crushed garlic
- sea salt and pepper to taste

Rinse swordfish and pat dry with paper towels. Place water in a stovetop pan with a steamer basket or inserted steamer. Heat water to boiling. Place swordfish in steamer and top with lemon juice, garlic, and salt and pepper. Steam until fish flakes easily with a fork, about 8-10 minutes.

Nutrition per serving: 138 calories; 4 g Total Fat; 1 g saturated fat; 22 g protein; 3 g carbohydrates; 0 g dietary fiber; 43 mg cholesterol; 377 mg sodium.

Pepita Coated Halibut

Coating the halibut with roasted pepitas adds zinc, an important mineral that helps to prevent cancer, lowers cholesterol, and promotes healthy skin and hair.

Makes 4 servings (serving = 1 filet)

- 4 (4 ounce) halibut filets
- ½ cup roasted pepitas, coarsely chopped
- ½ cup grated fresh parmesan cheese
- 2 cloves crushed garlic
- 1 teaspoon dried oregano
- 1 teaspoon cayenne pepper
- ½ cup oat flour
- 1 egg, whisked
- ½ cup coconut milk

Preheat oven to 350 degrees. Coat a baking dish with coconut oil. Combine pumpkin seeds, parmesan cheese, garlic, spices and oat flour in a shallow dish and mix well. Combine egg and coconut milk in a shallow dish and mix well. Dip each filet into the egg mixture, dredge through the pumpkin seed mixture on both sides and place in the baking dish. Bake uncovered for 20 minutes or until fish flakes easily with a fork.

Nutrition per serving: 389 calories; 22 g Total Fat; 10 g saturated fat; 36 g protein; 15 g carbohydrates; 3 g dietary fiber; 100 mg cholesterol; 435 mg sodium.

Grilled Marinated Salmon

The flavor of grilled salmon is delightful enough, and this marinade adds another dimension to its flavor.

Makes 4 servings (serving = 4 ounces salmon)

- ¼ cup wheat free tamari sauce, reduced sodium
- ¼ cup rice wine vinegar
- 1 tablespoon pure maple syrup (optional)
- 1 tablespoon coconut oil, liquid at room temperature
- 1 teaspoon dried mustard
- 1 teaspoon ground ginger
- 1 teaspoon ground black pepper
- 1 lb. salmon fillets

In a medium bowl, combine the soy sauce, vinegar, maple syrup, oil, dried mustard, ginger, and ground black pepper. Place the salmon in a shallow, nonporous dish and pour the marinade over the salmon. Cover and marinate in the refrigerator for at least 1 hour, turning occasionally. Preheat an outdoor grill at medium high heat and lightly oil grate. Grill the fish for about 3-4 minutes on each side, or to desired doneness.

Nutrition per serving: 229 calories; 13 g Total Fat; 5 g saturated fat; 24 g protein; 4 g carbohydrates; 0 g dietary fiber; 74 mg cholesterol; 221 mg sodium.

Charbroiled Salmon

There's just so many ways to enjoy salmon!

Makes 4 servings (serving = 4 ounces salmon)

- 1 cup wheat free tamari sauce, reduced sodium
- ½ teaspoon ground ginger
- ½ teaspoon ground black pepper
- 1 lb. salmon steaks
- 4 sprigs fresh parsley for garnish
- 4 slices lemon for garnish

Combine tamari sauce, ginger, and black pepper in a large, re-sealable plastic bag. Seal, and shake vigorously to mix ingredients. Add salmon steaks, squeeze out excess air, and seal. Refrigerate, turning frequently to keep all sides in contact with the liquid, for no less than 2 hours. Preheat an outdoor grill at medium high heat. Cook on a hot grill for about 5 minutes per side, basting freely with extra marinade. Serve with parsley garnish and lemon slices.

Nutrition per serving: 187 calories; 9 g Total Fat; 2 g saturated fat; 24 g protein; 2 g carbohydrates; 0 g dietary fiber; 74 mg cholesterol; 169 mg sodium.

Whole Grain Goodness

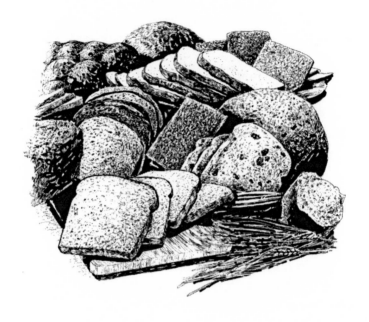

It's a mystery science has not been able to explain, but it's still true. All foods found in nature, when eaten in their natural whole state, contain all the corresponding nutrients and enzymes the human body requires to properly digest that particular food.

When we eat manipulated food like flour and sugar, we're eating a product that doesn't contain the nutrients necessary for the body to properly digest it – causing health problems down the road.

Plan-D Flourless Muffins™

This is the homemade version of my famous flourless oat bran muffins sold in natural food markets throughout the Southwest. You can exchange the raisins and walnuts for other fruits and nuts, or try replacing the applesauce with mashed bananas or pumpkin puree for different varieties.

Makes 1 dozen muffins (serving = 1 muffin)

Dry Ingredients:
- 2 cups raw oat bran
- 2 1/8 teaspoon baking powder
- 1 tablespoon cinnamon
- ½ teaspoon nutmeg
- ½ teaspoon sea salt

Wet Ingredients:
- 1 cup non-fat milk or unsweetened almond milk
- ½ cup unsweetened applesauce
- 2 large egg whites
- 1 teaspoon pure vanilla extract
- ½ teaspoon liquid stevia extract

Third Set of Ingredients:
- ½ cup raisins
- ½ cup walnuts, chopped
- ½ cup agave nectar or raw unfiltered honey

Preheat oven to 400 degrees. Line muffin pans with paper muffin cups or coat with coconut oil or butter.

Combine dry ingredients in a large mixing bowl and mix together thoroughly with a wire whisk. In a separate mixing bowl combine the wet ingredients with the wire whisk until the mixture becomes somewhat frothy. Slowly add wet ingredients to dry ingredients and mix thoroughly with a wooden spoon or use an electric mixer such as a Kitchen Aid. Fold in the raisins and walnuts. The last step is to add the agave or honey very slowly to the mixture while stirring. The batter should become lighter in texture.

Fill muffin cups and bake for 10 minutes at 400 degrees and then lower heat to 350 degrees. Bake for an additional 10 minutes, or until the muffins are golden brown and knife inserted in center comes out clean. Let cool in the pan.

Nutrition per serving: 126 calories; 5 g Total Fat; 0 g saturated fat; 5 g protein; 17 g carbohydrates; 4 g dietary fiber; 0 mg cholesterol; 180 mg sodium.

Perfect Cornbread

This golden cornbread is moist and lightly sweet. It's a delightful accompaniment to any meal.

Makes one 9x9x2 inch pan (about 8 pieces, serving = 1 piece)

- 1 cup whole wheat pastry flour
- 1 cup yellow corn meal
- ½ cup raw unfiltered honey
- 4 teaspoons baking powder
- ¾ teaspoon salt
- 2 eggs
- 1 cup nonfat milk, preferably organic
- ¼ cup butter, melted

Preheat oven to 425 degrees. Sift together flour, baking powder, and salt. Add cornmeal, eggs, and milk. Blend thoroughly. Stir in the melted butter and honey. Beat together until the batter is smooth. Pour batter into a 9x9x2 inch oiled pan, and bake for 20-25 minutes or until golden brown.

Nutrition per serving: 252 calories; 8 g Total Fat; 4 g saturated fat; 4 g protein; 41 g carbohydrates; 3 g dietary fiber; 69 mg cholesterol; 417 mg sodium

Southwest Blue-Green Cornbread

Blue corn contains much higher concentrations of iron, protein, and several other minerals than yellow or white corn, which makes it softer and less starchy. Because of its unique starch characteristics, blue cornmeal produces especially light and tender baked products.

Makes one 9x13 inch baking pan (about 16 pieces, serving = 1 piece)

- 1 cup whole wheat pastry flour
- 1 ¼ cups blue cornmeal
- ¼ teaspoon liquid stevia extract
- 1 teaspoon salt
- 1 tablespoon baking powder
- 2 tablespoons coconut oil
- 1 can (4 ounce) roasted green chilies
- 1 medium red bell pepper, seeded and diced
- 1 medium green bell pepper, seeded and diced
- 3 garlic cloves, minced
- 2 eggs
- 6 tablespoons coconut oil, melted and cooled
- 6 tablespoons unsalted butter, melted and cooled
- 1/8 teaspoon baking soda
- 1 cup nonfat buttermilk, at room temperature
- 3 tablespoons fresh cilantro, chopped

Preheat oven to 400 degrees. Butter a 9x13 inch baking pan. Sift together the flour, cornmeal, stevia, salt and baking powder. In a skillet over medium heat, sauté the bell peppers and garlic in the 2 tablespoons coconut oil until soft, about 4 minutes. Add the can of green chilies. Set aside.

In a large bowl, whisk the eggs and add the 6 tablespoons melted coconut oil and 6 tablespoons melted unsalted butter.

Stir the baking soda into the buttermilk and add it to the egg mixture. Add the dry ingredients, and mix well until the batter is just smooth; do not over mix. Fold in the vegetable mixture and cilantro.

Pour the batter into the prepared pan. Bake in the center of the oven for 25 to 30 minutes, or until the top is brown. Serve immediately. Store leftovers in the freezer for up to 3 months.

Nutrition per serving: 174 calories; 12 g Total Fat; 9 g saturated fat; 3 g protein; 14 g carbohydrates; 1 g dietary fiber; 38 mg cholesterol; 235 mg sodium

Flourless Herbed Croutons

Giving up flour doesn't mean giving up croutons. These are especially flavorful.

Makes 4 cups (serving = ¼ cup)

- 2 tablespoons extra virgin olive oil
- 2 teaspoons chopped fresh rosemary, oregano, basil, or thyme (or ½ teaspoon dried herbs)
- ½ teaspoon course sea salt
- 4 cups Ezekiel bread or other flourless sprouted grain bread, cut into cubes

Preheat oven to 350 degrees. In a large bowl, mix together oil, herbs, and sea salt; tilt the bowl to cover sides with oil mixture. Add the bread cubes and toss to coat. Spread in a single layer on ungreased baking sheet. Bake for about 20 minutes. Cool completely. Store in an airtight container.

Nutrition per serving: 30 calories; 2 g Total Fat; 0 g saturated fat; 1 g protein; 2 g carbohydrates; <1 g dietary fiber; 0 mg cholesterol; 103 mg sodium.

Flourless Herbed Stuffing

Great for Thanksgiving or any time of the year.

Makes 6 cups (serving = ½ cup)

- 3-4 cups Flourless Herbed Croutons (see index)
- 1 cup celery, chopped
- 1/3 cup onion, chopped
- ½ cup carrots, chopped
- ½ cup walnuts, chopped
- 1 tablespoon fresh parsley, chopped
- 4 cloves fresh garlic, minced
- 1 cup turkey, chicken, or vegetable stock, hot
- ¼ teaspoon black pepper
- ¼ teaspoon ground sage
- ¼ teaspoon dried marjoram
- ¼ teaspoon dried thyme
- 1//8 teaspoon dried basil
- coconut oil, for greasing the pan

Preheat oven to 350 degrees. Combine all ingredients in a large bowl. Toss with a wooden spoon. Pour the mixture into a casserole dish lightly oiled with coconut oil. Bake for 30-40 minutes. This recipe may also be used as a stuffing for turkey, chicken, and Cornish hens.

Nutrition per serving: 94 calories; 7 g Total Fat; 2 g saturated fat; 3 g protein; 5 g carbohydrates; 1 g dietary fiber; 0 mg cholesterol; 154 mg sodium.

Whole Grain Muffin Mix

Delicious whether freshly baked, reheated or toasted.

Makes 1 dozen muffins

- 1 cup whole wheat flour
- 1 cup spelt flour
- ½ cup oat bran
- ½ cup raw wheat germ
- ¼ cup rolled oats
- 1/3 cup ground flaxseeds
- ½ teaspoon baking soda
- 1 tablespoon baking powder
- ½ teaspoon sea salt

- ½ stick butter, melted
- 1/3 cup orange juice
- ¾ cup raisins

- 1 mashed banana
- 1 ¾ cup low fat milk or soy milk
- 1 beaten egg
- 1 tablespoon apple cider vinegar

- 1 cup chopped walnuts or pecans
- 2 teaspoons stevia concentrate

Preheat oven to 375 degrees. Line muffin pans with paper muffin cups or coat with coconut oil.

In a small pan, simmer the raisins and orange juice for 3-5 minutes. Add the butter and stir until it melts. Remove from heat and set aside.

In a large mixing bowl, combine oat bran, wheat germ, flours, baking powder, baking soda, and salt. Mix together well.

In a separate bowl, combine the milk, egg, mashed banana, and the raisin orange juice butter mixture. Add the dry ingredients to the wet and stir with a wooden spoon to combine. Add the stevia and nuts. Stir to mix thoroughly.

Fill muffin cups to almost overflowing and bake for 20 minutes, or until a knife inserted into the center of a muffin comes out clean. Cool on a wire rack.

Nutrition per serving: 293 calories; 13 g Total Fat; 4 g saturated fat; 8 g protein; 34 g carbohydrates; 5 g dietary fiber; 29 mg cholesterol; 237 mg sodium.

Vegetarian Delights

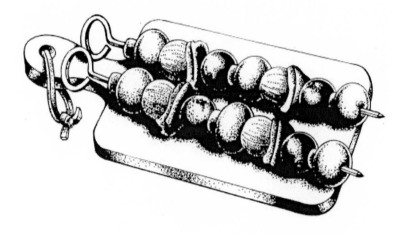

If you select your vegetables wisely, you can create a multivitamin out of your meal.

Veggie Shish Kabob

These kebobs have a wonderful peanutty flavor!

Makes 6 servings (serving = 1 skewer)

- 1 pound extra firm tofu, cut into ¾ inch cubes
- 6 cherry tomatoes
- 6 shallots, peeled
- 1/2 green bell pepper, cut into cubes
- 1/2 red bell pepper, cut into cubes
- 1/2 yellow bell pepper, cut into cubes
- 1 zucchini, sliced thickly
- 4 tablespoons low sodium tamari sauce
- 1 tablespoon toasted sesame oil
- 6 tablespoons mirin
- 2 tablespoons pure maple syrup
- 2 tablespoons natural peanut butter
- 6 wooden or metal skewers

Whisk together tamari sauce, mirin, maple syrup, peanut butter, and sesame oil in a bowl. Set aside.

Place tofu and vegetables on the skewers, alternating colors. Set shish kabobs in a shallow baking dish. Cover with the tamari sauce mixture, making sure tofu and vegetables are coated. Marinate for 1 hour. Place shish kabobs on a prepared grill or broil in the oven.

Nutrition per serving: 217 calories; 11 g Total Fat; 2 g saturated fat; 15 g protein; 13 g carbohydrates; <1 g dietary fiber; 0 mg cholesterol; 471 mg sodium.

Baked Sweet Potatoes

Sweet potatoes are high in vitamin A, lower in starch than white potatoes, and absolutely delicious.

Makes 4 servings (serving = 1 potato)

- 4 medium sweet potatoes, even in size (about 1 pound)
- 1 teaspoon butter, optional
- dash of paprika or cinnamon, optional

Heat oven to 450 degrees. Scrub potatoes. Arrange potatoes on oven rack and bake for 35 to 45 minutes, until tender. Remove and prick with a fork to let steam out. Cut a 1 ½ inch cross in the center of each potato. Hold each potato with potholders and press upward from the bottom until filling bursts through the cuts.

The great news about sweet potatoes is that they are very sweet and delicious eaten plain, just as they are.

If you must, top with butter and sprinkle with paprika or cinnamon.

Nutrition per serving: 130 calories; 1 g Total Fat; <1 g saturated fat; 2 g protein; 28 g carbohydrates; 1 g dietary fiber; 2 mg cholesterol; 24 mg sodium.

Mexican Eggplant Casserole

Mexican food is my favorite. This easy recipe blends the flavors from south of the border with eggplant, a highly nutritious vegetable.

Makes 8 servings
Serving size: 6 ounces

- 1 small eggplant (about 1 pound), peeled and cut into ½ inch cubes
- 4 corn tortillas
- 1 cup cheddar cheese, grated
- 1 (15 ounce) can chunky stewed tomatoes
- 1 teaspoon Mexican oregano
- 1 teaspoon cumin
- 1 teaspoon chili powder

Heat oven to 350 degrees. Place tortillas on oven rack and heat until golden brown and no longer pliable, approximately 3-5 minutes. Watch tortillas closely as they burn quickly. Allow tortillas to cool completely. Crumble tortillas into small pieces.

Empty the can of stewed tomatoes into a saucepan and heat over medium heat until just boiling. Add oregano, cumin, and chili powder, reduce heat and simmer 10 minutes. Remove from heat and set aside.

Coat a baking dish (8x8x2 inches) with coconut oil. Heat ½ inch water to boiling in a small saucepan. Add eggplant and return to boiling. Reduce heat to medium and cook 5 minutes; drain. Mix tortilla pieces and cheese. Spread half of the eggplant in the baking dish and spoon half of the tomato mixture over the eggplant. Sprinkle with half of the tortilla cheese mixture. Repeat layers with the remaining ingredients. Bake uncovered about 30 minutes or until bubbly around the edges.

Nutrition per serving: 145 calories; 6 g Total Fat; 3 g saturated fat; 5 g protein; 17 g carbohydrates; 2 g dietary fiber; 15 mg cholesterol; 103 mg sodium.

Easy Sautéed Greens

A flavorful twist on a southern tradition.

Makes 2 servings

- 1 tablespoon coconut oil
- 1 tablespoon toasted sesame oil (expeller pressed, unrefined)
- 2 cloves garlic, minced
- 1 tablespoon fresh ginger root, peeled and minced
- 1 bag (10 ounce) baby spinach or collard greens
- 1 tablespoon low sodium soy sauce
- 1 teaspoon sesame seeds, toasted (see note below)

Heat oils in a skillet over medium heat. Add garlic and ginger, cook, stirring until garlic softens, about 1 minute. Add greens; cook until leaves soften and heat through, 1-2 minutes. Add soy sauce and sesame seeds; toss to combine. Serve immediately.

Note: To toast sesame seeds, place them in a dry skillet over low heat, shaking frequently to prevent burning, until fragrant and barely colored, about 3 minutes or place in a shallow pan in a toaster oven and bake at 300 degrees for approximately 3-5 minutes.

Nutrition per serving: 172 calories; 14 g Total Fat; 7 g saturated fat; 5 g protein; 7 g carbohydrates; 1 g dietary fiber; 71 mg cholesterol; 449 mg sodium.

Baked Eggplant Parmesan

This is a flourless version of everyone's favorite Italian entrée.

Makes 8 servings (serving = 2 slices with sauce)

- 1 large eggplant
- 1 cup oat bran
- 1 cup grated parmesan cheese
- 2 eggs, whisked
- 2 cups Dee's No Sugar Marinara Sauce (see index)
- 1 cup shredded part skim mozzarella cheese

Peel eggplant and slice into 16, ¼ inch slices. Sprinkle with sea salt and place in a colander for about an hour to draw out moisture. Rinse eggplant slices and pat dry with paper towels. Preheat oven to 400 degrees.

Coat a large baking sheet with coconut oil. In a shallow bowl, combine oat bran and parmesan cheese. Place whisked eggs in another shallow dish. Dip each eggplant slice into eggs, coating both sides. Then dip into the oat bran mixture, also coating both sides. Place eggplant slices on the prepared baking sheet. Bake at 400 degrees for 25 minutes or until coating is golden brown.

Pour ½ of the marinara sauce in the baking dish and spread evenly to cover the bottom. Layer eggplant slices on top of the sauce, overlapping slightly if necessary. Top eggplant with remaining sauce and sprinkle with grated mozzarella cheese. Continue baking approximately 10 minutes or until sauce is heated and cheese is melted.

Nutrition per serving: 222 calories; 9 g Total Fat; 4 g saturated fat; 14 g protein; 20 g carbohydrates; 4 g dietary fiber; 71 mg cholesterol; 763 mg sodium.

Nuts About Tofu

Peanuts and tofu are two great source of vegetable protein.

Makes 4 servings

- 1 pound extra-firm tofu, drained and pressed for 15 minutes
- ½ cup coconut milk
- ¼ cup natural peanut butter, chunky
- ¼ teaspoon liquid stevia
- 1 ½ teaspoon low sodium wheat free tamari sauce
- 2 cloves fresh garlic, minced
- 1 teaspoon fresh ginger, peeled and minced
- 4 shallots, peeled and minced
- 6 green onions, sliced
- ¼ teaspoon cayenne pepper
- ½ cup dry roasted peanuts, unsalted

- 1 tablespoon coconut oil

Place coconut milk, peanut butter, stevia, and tamari sauce in a blender or food processor and puree until smooth. Set aside. Cut tofu into ¾ inch cubes. Heat oil over medium heat in a nonstick skillet. Brown the tofu in the oil, turning every 2-3 minutes (not all sides need to be brown). Add the garlic, ginger, and shallots and continue to cook until the shallots are translucent. Add the coconut milk mixture to the tofu and stir to coat. Reduce and simmer 10 minutes. Remove from heat. Transfer to a serving dish. Sprinkle with green onions and peanuts.

Nutrition per serving: 498 calories; 35 g Total Fat; 10 g saturated fat; 28 g protein; 16 g carbohydrates; 2 g dietary fiber; 0 mg cholesterol; 145 mg sodium.

Broccoli in Spicy Orange Sauce

Broccoli florets contain healthful nutrients such as vitamin C, calcium, folate and fiber. Add the orange sauce and you get an extra dose of vitamin C.

Makes 6 servings (serving = 1 cup)

- 2 tablespoons coconut oil
- 2 tablespoons toasted sesame oil
- 3 tablespoons soy sauce
  ½ cup orange juice
- 3 tablespoons water
- 1 tablespoon finely grated orange peel

- 2 garlic cloves, minced
- 4 cups broccoli florets
- 12 green onions, cut into small pieces
- ½ teaspoon ground ginger
- ¼ teaspoon crushed red pepper flakes
- 1 tablespoon arrowroot

In a small bowl, mix the arrowroot with the water until dissolved. Add soy sauce, orange juice, and orange peel; stir and set aside.

Heat the coconut oil over medium heat in a large skillet or wok. Sauté garlic for 30 seconds. Add broccoli, green onions, ginger, pepper flakes and sesame oil. Stir-fry for 2 minutes or until the broccoli is slightly tender. Add the orange juice mixture and stir for 2 more minutes or until the sauce is thickened. Serve over brown rice.

Nutrition per serving: 139 calories; 9 g Total Fat; 4 g saturated fat; 4 g protein; 11 g carbohydrates; 1 g dietary fiber; 0 mg cholesterol; 258 mg sodium.

Snow Peas with Cashews and Basil Vinaigrette

Presentation is everything. This dish appeals to the eye and the palate.

Makes 4 servings (serving = 1 cup)

- 1 tablespoon apple cider vinegar
- 1 tablespoon fresh basil, finely chopped
- dash of Herbamare
- 4 tablespoons extra virgin olive oil
- ½ cup drained bottled whole roasted red pepper, cut into strips
- 8 ounces fresh snow peas, trimmed and strings discarded
- 2 tablespoons raw cashews, finely chopped

In a small bowl, whisk together the vinegar, basil, and Herbamare to taste. Add the olive oil in a stream, whisking until the dressing is emulsified. Add the red pepper strips and let them marinate in the dressing for 10 minutes.

Blanch the snow peas by placing them in boiling water for 10 seconds, drain them and then plunge into a bowl of ice cold water. Drain and pat dry. Drain the red pepper strips, reserving all the dressing.

On a large plate or platter, decoratively arrange the snow peas and red pepper strips. Whisk the dressing and drizzle it over the vegetables. Top with chopped cashews.

Nutrition per serving: 168 calories; 15 g Total Fat; 2 g saturated fat; 2 g protein; 7 g carbohydrates; 2 g dietary fiber; 0 mg cholesterol; 332 mg sodium.

Creamy Spaghetti Squash
With Asparagus and Rosemary

Try this instead of eating pasta.

Makes 4 servings (serving = 1 cup)

- 1 small spaghetti squash
- 1 tablespoon extra virgin olive oil
- 1 pound thin asparagus, steamed tender
- 4 cloves fresh garlic, minced
- 1 tablespoon fresh rosemary, chopped
- dash of Herbamare
- 1 tablespoon coconut oil
- 1 cup part skim ricotta cheese
- 1 tablespoon toasted pine nuts

Heat oven to 350 degrees. Fill a baking dish with about ½ inch of water. Cut the squash in half and place it face down in the baking dish. Bake in the oven until done, about 30 minutes or until tender when tested with a fork. Throw away the seeds.

Scrape out the squash with a fork and place the stringy squash in a mixing bowl. Drizzle with the olive oil, and season with Herbamare.

Heat the coconut oil in a large nonstick skillet over medium heat. Slice asparagus into 1-inch pieces and sauté them with the garlic and rosemary for 1 minute. Stir in 1 cup ricotta and squash. Sauté until hot and creamy. Top with 1 tablespoon pine nuts.

Nutrition per serving: 355 calories; 15 g Total Fat; 7 g saturated fat; 14 g protein; 40 g carbohydrates; 8 g dietary fiber; 19 mg cholesterol; 485 mg sodium.

Grilled Vegetable Frittata

This is great for breakfast, lunch, or dinner.

Makes 4 servings (serving = ¼ of frittata)

- 2 tablespoons coconut oil
- 1 medium onion, chopped
- 1 yellow bell pepper
- 1 green bell pepper
- 6 asparagus spears, cut into 1 inch pieces
- 1 zucchini sliced
- 1 tablespoon fresh basil
- 3 cloves fresh garlic, minced
- 8 large eggs
- 1 cup lite coconut milk
- ½ cup grated organic cheddar cheese or almond cheese (optional)
- salt and ground black pepper to taste

Heat oil in a large skillet over medium heat. Sauté the bell peppers asparagus, and onion until they are tender. Add zucchini, stir and cook until heated through. Stir in basil and garlic. Set aside.

Crack the eggs into a large mixing bowl. Add the coconut milk and the salt and pepper and whisk. Place the vegetables into a lightly—oiled shallow baking dish and pour the egg mixture over them. Sprinkle with the cheese. Bake at 350 degrees for about 25 minutes, until puffed and golden.

Nutrition per serving: 406 calories; 29 g Total Fat; 16 g saturated fat; 24 g protein; 12 g carbohydrates; 1 g dietary fiber; 610 mg cholesterol; 574 mg sodium.

Steamed Vegetable Medley

A medley of steamed veggies in a light olive oil seasoning.

Makes 4 servings (serving = 1 cup)

- 1 cup broccoli florets
- 1 cup carrots, sliced diagonal
- ½ cup zucchini, sliced
- ½ cup yellow squash, sliced
- 1 cup fresh green beans
- 1 teaspoon dried basil
- 1 tablespoon extra virgin olive oil

Place broccoli, carrots, and green beans in a steamer basket. Cover and steam vegetables for 10-15 minutes. Add zucchini and yellow squash, sprinkle with basil, and steam 2 minutes more. Transfer vegetables to a bowl and toss with olive oil. Serve immediately.

Nutrition per serving: 65 calories; 3 g Total Fat; 0 g saturated fat; 2 g protein; 7 g carbohydrates; 1 g dietary fiber; 0 mg cholesterol; 102 mg sodium.

Steamed Brown Rice

Brown rice is more dense than white rice and typically has a longer simmer time.

Makes 4 servings

- 1 cup brown basmati rice or short grain brown rice
- 1 ½ to 2 cups water

Combine water and rice in a saucepan. Bring to a boil over high heat. Let boil for 5 minutes, stirring occasionally. Reduce heat to simmer, cover pan, and allow rice to cook slowly until all water has been absorbed, approximately 50-60 minutes. Do not stir the rice after you have lowered the heat and covered the pan.

Hint: A rice cooker or a steamer that has a rice cooking feature is a handy kitchen tool. Follow manufacturer directions for rice cooking times.

Nutrition per serving: 108 calories; <1 g Total Fat; 0 g saturated fat; 2 g protein; 23 g carbohydrates; <1 g dietary fiber; 0 mg cholesterol; 1 mg sodium.

Butternut Brown Rice

If you don't know what to do with butternut squash, throw it into the rice!

Makes 4 servings (serving = 1 cup)

- 1 tablespoon coconut oil
- 2 cloves fresh garlic, peeled and minced
- 1 cup onion, finely chopped
- 3 cups low sodium fat-free chicken broth
- 1 medium yellow bell pepper, stemmed, seeded and finely chopped
- 1 cup butternut squash, cut into ½ inch cubes
- 1 medium tomato, coarsely chopped
- 1 teaspoon ground cumin
- ½ teaspoon chili powder
- 1 cup basmati brown rice
- 1 tablespoon slivered almonds
- 2 tablespoons fresh parsley, minced

Heat oil over medium heat in a large nonstick skillet. Add the garlic, yellow bell pepper and onion and sauté 3 minutes. Add the chicken broth, rice, squash, tomato, cumin, and chili powder and stir. Bring the rice to a boil for 5 minutes stirring frequently. Reduce heat, cover and let simmer for 35-40 minutes. Remove from heat and stir in the parsley and almonds. Replace cover and let sit 5 minutes. Serve hot.

Nutrition per serving: 182 calories; 5 g Total Fat; 3 g saturated fat; 6 g protein; 29 g carbohydrates; 1 g dietary fiber; 0 mg cholesterol; 55 mg sodium.

Eastern Quinoa Pilaf

Quinoa is a gluten free whole grain. It contains more protein than any other grain.

Makes 4 servings (serving = ½ cup)

- 1 cup fat-free chicken broth
- 1 cup water
- 1 cup quinoa
- ¼ teaspoon ground cloves
- 1 bay leaf
- ½ teaspoon ground cardamom
- ¼ teaspoon ground cinnamon
- ½ cup frozen green peas
- ½ cup carrots, finely chopped

Place quinoa, water, and chicken broth in a medium saucepan and bring to a boil. Add peas, carrots, cloves, bay leaf, cardamom, and cinnamon. Let boil for 5 minutes. Reduce heat, cover, and simmer until all the liquid is absorbed, about 10-15 minutes. When done, the quinoa appears soft and translucent. Remove bay leaf, fluff with a fork, and serve.

Nutrition per serving: 192 calories; 3 g Total Fat; <1 g saturated fat; 7 g protein; 34 g carbohydrates; 3 g dietary fiber; 0 mg cholesterol; 51 mg sodium

Sesame Brown Rice

This is a flavorful variation for cooking brown rice.

Makes 4 servings (serving = ½ cup)

- 1 cup brown basmati rice
- 1 ½ cups water or low sodium chicken or vegetable broth
- 1 tablespoon reduced sodium soy sauce or wheat-free tamari sauce
- 1 tablespoon toasted sesame oil (expeller pressed, unrefined)
- 2 teaspoons toasted sesame seeds
- 1 tablespoon chopped green onions (green parts only)

Bring water or broth and rice to a boil for 5 minutes. Add, soy sauce and sesame oil. Cover and simmer for 40-50 minutes or until liquid is absorbed. Fluff with fork and garnish with onions and sesame seeds.

To toast sesame seeds, place them in a dry skillet over low heat, shaking frequently to prevent burning, until fragrant and barely colored, about 3 minutes.

Note: Use quick cooking brown rice, if desired. Adjust cooking time according to package instructions.

Nutrition per serving: 146 calories; 4 g Total Fat; <1 g saturated fat; 3 g protein; 24 g carbohydrates; <1 g dietary fiber; 0 mg cholesterol; 178 mg sodium

"Refried" Pinto Beans

This version of refried beans has no fat whatsoever!

Makes 6 servings (serving = ½ cup)

- 1 pound dried pinto beans
- 3 quarts water
- 1 medium onion, finely chopped
- 3 cloves garlic, minced
- 2 teaspoons ground cumin
- 2 teaspoons Mexican oregano
- 2 teaspoons salt

Place beans in a stock pot and cover with water. Let soak overnight. Drain the beans and rinse thoroughly. Place the beans back into the stock pot, add 3 quarts water and spices. Stir. Bring to a boil. Reduce heat to medium, but allow the beans to gently boil. Stir frequently. Add more water if necessary. Do not let the water get too low. Beans are done when speckles are no longer visible and they turn dark brown.

Drain beans and reserve the hot liquid. Place beans in a large mixing bowl. Add a small amount of the reserved liquid. Mix with an electric mixer, adding liquid until the beans have a smooth creamy consistency. Serve hot.

Nutrition per serving: 143 calories; 0 g Total Fat; 0 g saturated fat; 8 g protein; 27 g carbohydrates; 3 g dietary fiber; 0 mg cholesterol; 275 mg sodium

Dee's No Sugar Marinara Sauce

I gave up eating the pasta, but not the sauce! This is great on steamed veggies, baked potatoes, and Eggplant Parmesan.

Makes 4 cups (serving = ½ cup)

- 1 can (28 ounce) diced tomatoes, including liquid
- 2 cans (8 ounce) tomato sauce
- 1 can (6 ounce) tomato paste
- 2 cups water
- 2 bay leaves
- 2 teaspoons dried basil
- 2 teaspoons dried parsley
- 2 teaspoons dried oregano
- 2 teaspoons ground sage
- 1 teaspoon dried rosemary
- 1 teaspoon dried thyme
- 1 teaspoon sea salt
- 4 cloves fresh garlic, minced
- 1 onion, finely chopped
- 1 tablespoon extra virgin olive oil
- 1 tablespoon coconut oil

Heat coconut oil over medium heat in a large stock pot. Add garlic and onions and sauté until translucent. Add diced tomatoes with liquid, tomato sauce, tomato paste, and spices. Bring to a boil. Reduce heat and let simmer to up to 1 hour, adding water if necessary. Serve immediately or store in an airtight container.

Nutrition per serving: 109 calories; 2 g Total Fat; 1 g saturated fat; 3 g protein; 19 g carbohydrates; 2 g dietary fiber; 0 mg cholesterol; 320 mg sodium

Thyme Roasted Vegetables

Roasted vegetables are always a treat. The natural sugar in the vegetables caramelizes during roasting and creates an incredibly sweet-savory flavor.

Makes 8 servings (serving = ½ cup)

- 8 ounces shallots, peeled
- 2 medium red-skinned potatoes, cut into 1 ½ inch pieces
- 2 medium parsnips, peeled and cut into 1 ½ inch pieces
- 4 medium carrots, cut into 1 ½ inch pieces
- 1 small rutabaga, peeled and cut into 1 ½ inch pieces
- 4 cloves garlic, minced
- ¼ cup coconut oil, liquid at room temperature
- 1 tablespoon fresh thyme, chopped
- thyme sprigs for garnish
- sea salt and pepper to taste

Preheat oven to 450 degrees. In a large bowl, combine the vegetables, garlic, oil, thyme, salt and pepper. Toss to coat the vegetables evenly.

Transfer coated vegetables to a large baking dish and bake until tender and browned, 35 to 40 minutes. Serve hot.

Nutrition per serving: 211 calories; 7 g Total Fat; 6 g saturated fat; 4 g protein; 33 g carbohydrates; 3 g dietary fiber; 0 mg cholesterol; 182 mg sodium

Savvy Sandwiches &
Savory Soups

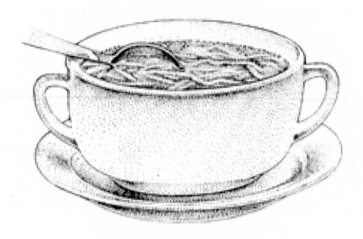

*A soup can be the highlight of a meal when it's filled with
fresh vegetables, legumes, and whole grains.*

Garden Vegetable Soup

Loaded with antioxidants, this soup is great for strengthening your immune system.

Makes 8 servings (serving = 1 cup)

- 2/3 cup sliced carrot
- ½ cup diced onion
- 2 garlic cloves, minced
- 3 cups fat-free chicken or vegetable broth
- 1 can (15 ounce) diced tomatoes with juice
- 1 ½ cups diced green cabbage
- ½ cup green beans, fresh or frozen
- 1 tablespoon tomato paste
- 1 teaspoon dried basil
- ½ teaspoon dried oregano
- ½ teaspoon sea salt
- ½ cup diced zucchini
- 1 tablespoon coconut oil
- water as needed

In a large stockpot, heat the coconut oil over medium heat and sauté the carrot, onion, and garlic until softened, about 5 minutes.

Add broth, diced tomatoes with juice, tomato paste, green beans, basil, oregano, and salt. Bring to a boil. Lower heat and simmer, covered, about 15 minutes or until green beans are tender. Add water if needed.

Stir in cabbage and zucchini and heat 3-4 minutes more. Serve hot.

Nutrition per serving: 55 calories; 2 g Total Fat; 1 g saturated fat; 2 g protein; 7 g carbohydrates; 2 g dietary fiber; 0 mg cholesterol; 201 mg sodium

Variations: Add other vegetables such as broccoli, cauliflower, corn, lima beans, spinach, etc. Also, add kidney beans or barley.

For extra immune strengthening, add astragalus root to the soup while cooking.

Savory Split Pea Soup

My vegetarian clients rave about this soup because it's loaded with flavor without adding ham.

Makes 8 servings (serving = 1 cup)

- 8 cups water
- 1 pound dried green split peas, sorted and rinsed
- 3 medium carrots, sliced thickly (1 ½ cups)
- 2 medium stalks celery, chopped (1 cup)
- 1 medium onion, chopped (1/2 cup)
- 2 cloves fresh garlic, minced
- 2 bay leaves
- 1 teaspoon sea salt
- 1 teaspoon dried thyme leaves
- 1 teaspoon dried basil
- 1 teaspoon dried oregano
- 1 teaspoon dried rosemary
- ¼ teaspoon black pepper

Mix all ingredients in a large stock pot and bring to a boil. Reduce heat to medium and simmer until done, about 1 ½ hours. Stir and add water as needed.

Nutrition per serving: 232 calories; <1 g Total Fat; 0 g saturated fat; 15 g protein; 41 g carbohydrates; 3 g dietary fiber; 0 mg cholesterol; 309 mg sodium

Barley Soup with Mushrooms and Root Vegetables

Barley is a whole grain that does not get enough attention, nor do we eat enough of it.

Makes 6 servings (serving = 1 ½ cups)

- 3 tablespoons coconut oil
- 1 medium onion, diced
- 2 cloves garlic, minced
- 1 large or 2 small ribs celery, leaves included, chopped
- 2 medium carrots, thickly sliced
- 1 medium parsnip, finely chopped
- 1 medium rutabaga, finely chopped
- 1 pound fresh mushrooms, coarsely chopped
- ½ teaspoon sea salt
- 1 teaspoon dried thyme
- 1 teaspoon dried sage
- 1 bay leaf
- ½ teaspoon freshly ground pepper
- 2/3 cup quick-cooking barley

- 1 quart low sodium chicken or vegetable broth
- 4 cups water

Heat oil in large stockpot over medium heat. Add onion, garlic, celery, parsnip, and rutabaga to the pot. Add a small amount of chicken broth. Chop mushrooms coarsely and add to the pot along with salt, thyme, sage, and pepper. Increase heat to medium high and cook, stirring, for about 5 minutes. Mushrooms should shrink considerably and get quite dark. Add chicken broth, water, and bay leaf and bring to a boil. Reduce heat to low and simmer for 20 minutes. Add barley and simmer 10 minutes longer or until barley is tender. Serve hot.

Nutrition per serving: 237 calories; 8 g Total Fat; 6 g saturated fat; 7 g protein; 35 g carbohydrates; 3 g dietary fiber; 0 mg cholesterol; 282 mg sodium

Carrot Ginger Soup

Carrots and ginger help rejuvenate the pancreas, the main organ responsible for regulating blood sugar levels.

Makes 8 servings (serving = ½ cup)

- 2 tablespoons coconut oil
- 2 small yellow onions, peeled and diced
- 2-3 cloves fresh garlic, crushed
- 2 pounds (16 medium) carrots, peeled and diced
- 3 tablespoons chopped scallions

- 1 tablespoon minced fresh ginger
- 3 cups fat-free chicken or vegetable broth
- ½ cup coconut milk
- sea salt and toasted crushed peppercorns to taste

Heat oil over medium heat in a stockpot. Sauté onions, garlic, carrots, scallions, and ginger over medium heat about 10 minutes. Add broth, bring to boil and simmer for 5 minutes. Transfer the soup to a food processor and puree in batches until smooth. Pour it back into the stockpot and stir in the coconut milk. Bring to a slow simmer but do not boil. Season to taste with salt and crushed peppercorns.

Remove from heat and serve.

Nutrition per serving: 174 calories; 9 g Total Fat; 6 g saturated fat; 3 g protein; 20 g carbohydrates; 2 g dietary fiber; 0 mg cholesterol; 222 mg sodium

Francene's Fabulous Lentil Soup

Lentils are very low in fat, high in fiber and are frequently referred to as a wonder food for their health promoting qualities.

Makes 8 servings (serving = 1 cup)

- 1 tablespoon coconut oil
- 1 tablespoon butter
- 2 celery stalks, diced

- 1 onion, peeled and chopped
- 2 cloves fresh garlic, chopped
- 2 carrots, diced
- 1 teaspoon dried basil
- ½ teaspoon celery seed
- 1 ½ tablespoon chopped fresh parsley
- 6-8 cups fat-free chicken or vegetable broth (or combo)
- 1 cup lentils
- ½ cup quick-cooking barley

Heat oil and butter over medium heat in a large stockpot. Sauté celery, onion, and garlic for three minutes. Add carrot; cover and cook for an additional three minutes.

Add broth, lentils, basil, celery seed, and parsley. Cook for two hours partially covered over low heat.

Add barley and cook an additional 15 minutes. Serve hot.

Nutrition per serving: 152 calories; 4 g Total Fat; 2 g saturated fat; 6 g protein; 24 g carbohydrates; 3 g dietary fiber; 4 mg cholesterol; 289 mg sodium

Special thanks to Francene Adcock, my partner in health, for contributing this recipe.

Zanzibar Roasted Vegetable Sandwich

This sandwich was inspired by one of my favorite menu items at Zanzibar, a great little coffee house in Pacific Beach, CA.

Makes 2 servings

- 4 slices Ezekial bread, toasted
- 1 tablespoon coconut oil
- 4 slices eggplant
- 1 red bell pepper, quartered
- ½ ripe avocado
- 2 slices provolone or jack cheese
- Handful of organic baby greens or spring mix
- 1 tablespoon lite safflower mayonnaise

Preheat oven to 425 degrees. Place eggplant slices and bell pepper in a shallow baking dish and coat with coconut oil. Roast in the oven for 10 minutes or until egg plant and bell pepper are soft. Remove the vegetables from the oven and reduce oven temperature to 300 degrees.

Place 2 eggplant slices, 2 quarters of the bell pepper, ¼ avocado, and one slice of cheese on one side of the toasted bread. Repeat for the other sandwich. Place the sandwich halves on a baking sheet and heat in the oven at 300 degrees until cheese is melted. Remove from oven and place on plates. Top with a handful of greens. Spread mayonnaise on the other piece of bread and place on top of the sandwich. Slice in half. Serve with a baby greens salad or bowl of Vegetable soup.

VARIATION: Add sliced turkey.

Nutrition per serving: 377 calories; 22 g Total Fat; 11 g saturated fat; 19 g protein; 27 g carbohydrates; 10 g dietary fiber; 20 mg cholesterol; 578 mg sodium

The Healthiest Tuna Fish Sandwich

Served with a nice green salad or a bowl of vegetable soup, this meal assures you get plenty of vegetables!

Makes 1 serving

- 2/3 cup Tasty Tuna Salad (see index)
- 2 slices Ezekiel Bread or other flourless bread, toasted
- ¼ ripe avocado, peeled and sliced
- 1 tomato slice
- 2 thin slices zucchini
- 2 romaine lettuce leaves or handful of spring mix

Place the tuna salad on one slice of the toasted bread. Top with tomato slice, 3 zucchini slices, avocado slices, and lettuce or spring mix. Place the second piece of toasted bread on top. Slice sandwich in half and serve.

Nutrition per serving: 379 calories; 17 g Total Fat; 2 g saturated fat; 32 g protein; 27 g carbohydrates; 9 g dietary fiber; 0 mg cholesterol; 353 mg sodium

Beti's Delight

This is a very nutritious snack or lunch idea. Be sure to complement it with an assortment of raw veggies such as baby carrots, cucumbers, and jicama.

Makes 2 servings

- 2/3 cup Tasty Tuna Salad (see index)
- 2 tablespoons low fat cottage cheese
- 1 Sprouted Grain English Muffin, split in half

Preheat oven or toaster oven to 350 degrees.

Mix tuna salad with cottage cheese. Put half of the mixture on each English muffin half and bake to heat; flip switch to "broil" to brown.

Variation: Add chopped black olives after it's broiled.

Many thanks to Beti Schwartz, one of my nutrition students, for contributing this recipe.

Nutrition per serving: 195 calories; 6 g Total Fat; 0 g saturated fat; 16 g protein; 19 g carbohydrates; 3 g dietary fiber; 1 mg cholesterol; 218 mg sodium

Asian Lettuce Wraps

*Lettuce wraps have become popular in Asian restaurants.
Now you can make them at home!*

Makes 4 servings

- 1 pound boneless chicken breasts, diced very small
- 16 Boston, Bibb or Butter lettuce leaves
- 1 can (8 ounce) sliced water chestnuts
- 1 large onion (for about 1 cup chopped)
- 2 tablespoons minced garlic
- 1 tablespoon reduced sodium wheat free tamari sauce
- ¼ cup hoisin sauce
- 2 teaspoons finely minced ginger
- 1 tablespoon Mirin
- ½ teaspoon red pepper flakes
- 1 bunch scallions (for about ¾ cup sliced)
- 2 teaspoons toasted sesame oil (unrefined, expeller pressed)

Rinse lettuce leaves, making sure to leave them whole, and set them aside to drain in a colander or on paper towels. Drain the water chestnuts, and finely chop them. Set aside.

Cook chicken in a 12 inch skillet over medium high heat. While the chicken cooks, peel and chop the onion and add to the chicken. Reduce heat to medium, stir frequently while adding the garlic, tamari sauce, hoisin sauce, ginger, vinegar and chili pepper sauce. Cook until chicken is done, about 10 minutes.

Add the water chestnuts. Rinse scallions and trim away the roots. Thinly slice scallions and add to the skillet. Add toasted sesame oil. Stir and cook just until the scallions begin to wilt, about 2 minutes. Remove from heat.

Arrange lettuce leaves around outer edge of serving platter. Pour the chicken mixture into the middle of the platter. To serve, allow each person to spoon some of the chicken mixture into the middle of each lettuce leaf and wrap the leaf around the chicken, taco style.

Nutrition per serving: 261 calories; 6 g Total Fat; 1 g saturated fat; 32 g protein; 20 g carbohydrates; 1 g dietary fiber; 77 mg cholesterol; 677 mg sodium

Tuna Salad Lettuce Wraps

This is a bread-free variation on the tuna sandwich.

Makes 1 serving

- 1 serving Tasty Tuna Salad (see index)
- 4 Romaine or Boston lettuce leaves
- ¼ ripe avocado, peeled and sliced
- 2 tomato slices, cut in half
- 4 thin slices zucchini
- 2 tomato slices, cut in half
- Handful of sprouts

Place the tuna salad on one leaf of lettuce. Add tomato, zucchini avocado, and sprouts. Roll up and eat. Repeat with remaining lettuce leaves.

Nutrition per serving: 433 calories; 28 g Total Fat; 3 g saturated fat; 27 g protein; 18 g carbohydrates; 4 g dietary fiber; 0 mg cholesterol; 112 mg sodium

Southwest Sensations

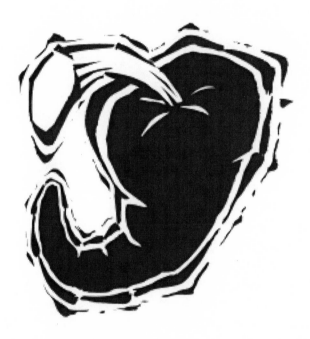

The main spices in southwestern food—cumin, cilantro, and cayenne pepper—raise your body temperature and can boost your metabolism. Studies show that these seasonings triple the body's ability to burn calories for fuel rather than store them as fat.

Turkey Chili & Beans

Beans are one of the most nutritious foods we can eat. They're high in fiber and a rich source of vegetarian protein.

Makes 8 servings (serving = 1 cup)

- 1 pound lean ground turkey
- 1 red onion, chopped
- 1 green bell pepper, chopped
- 1 yellow bell pepper, chopped
- 1 cup chopped carrots
- 5 cloves fresh garlic, minced
- 1 can (15 ounce) diced tomatoes, including liquid
- 1 can (8 ounce) reduced sodium tomato sauce
- 1 can (6 ounce) tomato paste
- 2 cups water
- 3 tablespoons chili powder
- 1 teaspoon dried Mexican oregano
- 2 teaspoons ground cumin
- 2 cans (15 ounce) pinto beans, rinsed and drained
- 1 can (15 ounce) red kidney beans, rinsed and drained

Place ground turkey, onion, and garlic in a large stockpot and cook over medium heat until the turkey is cooked through. Add carrots, bell peppers, stewed tomatoes, tomato paste, tomato sauce, and water. Increase heat to medium high until the mixture starts to boil. Add chili powder, oregano, cumin and beans. Reduce heat to medium and simmer 45 minutes, stirring occasionally. Serve with a fresh spring mix salad.

Refrigerate the leftover chili to eat the next day. It tastes even better when the spices have released their flavor overnight!

Nutrition per serving: 363 calories; 5 g Total Fat; <1 g saturated fat; 27 g protein; 54 g carbohydrates; 24 g dietary fiber; 33 mg cholesterol; 118 mg sodium

Southwestern White Chili

Canned beans are just as healthy as dried. When using beans canned in water (brine), rinse well under cold running water before adding to your recipe.

Makes 4 servings (serving = 1 cup)

- 1 tablespoon coconut oil
- 1 ½ pound boneless, skinless chicken breast, cut into small cubes
- ¼ cup chopped onion
- 1 cup chicken broth
- 1 can (4 ounce) chopped green chilies
- 2 green onions, sliced
- 1 can (19 ounce) white kidney beans (cannelloni), drained
- 1 teaspoon garlic powder
- ½ teaspoon ground red pepper
- 1 teaspoon ground cumin
- ½ teaspoon oregano leaves
- ½ teaspoon cilantro

Heat oil in a large saucepan over medium high heat. Add chicken and onions; cook 4 to 5 minutes.

Stir in broth, green chilies and spices, simmer 15 minutes.

Stir in beans. Simmer 5 minutes. Top with onions.

Nutrition per serving: 335 calories; 9 g Total Fat; 4 g saturated fat; 49 g protein; 14 g carbohydrates; 5 g dietary fiber; 116 mg cholesterol; 122 mg sodium

Robust Tortilla Soup

It's yummy and filling! Serve with a nice colorful salad. Garlic, cumin, and cilantro are metabolism boosting herbs and spices! Add them to your food as much as possible!

Makes 3 servings (serving = 1 ½ cups)

- 4 cups low sodium vegetable broth or fat-free chicken broth
- 2 boneless, skinless chicken breasts, cut into small chunks (about 8 ounces)
- 1 cup chopped tomatoes
- 1 tablespoon fresh squeezed lime juice
- 2 teaspoons chili powder
- 2 teaspoons ground cumin
- 2 cloves minced garlic
- 1 can (4 ounce) chopped green chilies
- 1 ripe avocado, diced and divided into three portions
- 3 servings baked tortilla chips (about 1 ounce each)
- ½ cup chopped cilantro
- 1 ounce shredded jack cheese (optional)

Cut up chicken into small chunks and place in a skillet with a small amount of the broth and the garlic. Add the chili powder and cumin and cook until the chicken is done.

Heat the rest of the broth in a large saucepan, and add the tomatoes and lime juice.

When the broth boils, lower heat. Add the chicken mixture and chilies and simmer for 5 minutes. Remove from heat. Spoon into bowls. To each bowl add tortilla chips, avocado, cheese, and cilantro. Serve hot.

Nutrition per serving: 429 calories; 18 g Total Fat; 4 g saturated fat; 29 g protein; 37 g carbohydrates; 4 g dietary fiber; 60 mg cholesterol; 611 mg sodium

Lasagna Mexicana

This recipe blends the idea of lasagna with the flavors of Mexico. Stone ground corn tortillas replace noodles for a flourless entrée.

Makes 8 servings (serving = 1/8 of casserole dish)

- 1 tablespoon coconut oil
- 1 onion, chopped
- 2 cloves garlic, minced
- 1 green bell pepper, chopped coarsely
- 1 pound ground turkey
- ½ teaspoon sea salt
- ½ teaspoon black pepper
- 1 teaspoon ground cumin
- 1 tablespoon chili powder or to taste
- Dash cayenne pepper (optional)
- 1 cup whole kernel corn (frozen or canned)
- One 15-ounce can pinto beans, drained
- One 15-ounce can dark red kidney beans, drained
- One 6-ounce can tomato paste
- One 8-ounce can tomato sauce
- One cup diced tomatoes
- One can (4 ounce) chopped mild green chilies
- Six 6-inch corn tortillas
- 1 cup cottage cheese
- ½ cup cheddar cheese, shredded

Preheat oven to 350 degrees. In a large skillet, heat the coconut oil over medium heat and sauté the onion, bell pepper and garlic until softened, about 5 minutes. Add in the ground turkey or ground beef. Stir in the spices and cook until meat is done. Remove from the heat. Mix in the green chilies, corn, beans, tomatoes, tomato paste and tomato sauce.

Coat a 2 or 3 -quart casserole dish with coconut oil. Place 3 tortillas in the 2-quart casserole dish, arranging them to cover the bottom. Spoon in half the meat mixture and spread ½ cup cottage cheese on top. Sprinkle on half the cheddar. Repeat layers using up all the ingredients. Bake covered at 350 degrees for 30-35 minutes. Let sit 5 minutes before serving.

Nutrition per serving: 417 calories; 7 g Total Fat; <1 g saturated fat; 27 g protein; 60 g carbohydrates; 15 g dietary fiber; 33 mg cholesterol; 253 mg sodium.

Tomato Lime Salsa

This chunky salsa adds flavor to steamed vegetables, omelets, and fish or poultry.

Makes 1 ½ cups, about 5 servings (serving = ½ cup)

- 1 cup seeded and finely chopped plum or Roma tomatoes
- ½ cup peeled, seeded and finely chopped cucumber
- 1 tablespoon finely chopped and seeded jalapeno pepper
- 1 tablespoon lime zest
- 2 teaspoons finely chopped garlic
- 3 tablespoons finely chopped fresh cilantro
- 1 ½ tablespoons chopped fresh mint
- ¼ teaspoon sea salt or to taste
- ¼ teaspoon black pepper or to taste

Place all ingredients in a glass or ceramic bowl and mix well. Let stand for 30 minutes. Taste and add more salt and pepper if needed. Salsa can be made a day ahead, covered and refrigerated.

To serve, drain salsa well and bring to room temperature before serving on grilled chicken or fish.

Nutrition per serving: 16 calories; 0 g Total Fat; 0 g saturated fat; <1 g protein; 3 g carbohydrates; 0 g dietary fiber; 0 mg cholesterol; 143 mg sodium.

Turkey and Black Bean Wraps

Great for that leftover Thanksgiving Day turkey.

Makes 4 wraps

- 2 medium tomatoes, chopped
- 1 cup canned black beans, rinsed and drained
- 1 can (4 ounce) diced green chilies
- 1/3 cup sliced green onions
- 2 tablespoons chopped fresh cilantro
- 1 tablespoon chili powder
- 1 teaspoon ground cumin
- ½ cup water
- 3 cups shredded cooked turkey
- 1 ripe avocado, quartered
- 3 cups shredded romaine lettuce
- 4 Ezekiel flourless sprouted grain tortillas

In a medium bowl, combine tomatoes, black beans, chiles, green onions and cilantro, set aside. In a large skillet, add water and spices. Mix and bring to a boil. Stir in turkey and reduce heat to low. Mix in tomato mixture and cook on low for 5 minutes, stirring occasionally. Scoop ¼ of the filling on to each tortilla. Top with lettuce and avocado quarters. Fold in sides and roll up to enclose filling.

Nutrition per serving: 457 calories; 14 g Total Fat; 3 g saturated fat; 37 g protein; 46 g carbohydrates; 9 g dietary fiber; 42 mg cholesterol; 331 mg sodium.

Black-Eyed Pea Enchiladas

Not all corn tortillas are created equal. Please check ingredient lists for added preservatives. Stone ground corn tortillas should only contain ground corn and lime.

Makes 8 servings (serving = 1 enchiladas)

- 1 medium white onion, diced (about 1 cup)
- 4 cloves fresh garlic, peeled and minced
- 2 tablespoons coconut oil
- 2 tablespoons chili powder
- ½ teaspoon dried oregano
- ½ teaspoon ground cumin
- ½ teaspoon sea salt
- ½ teaspoon crushed red pepper flakes
- 1 can (4 ounce) sliced black olives
- 2 cups organic black-eyed peas
- 8 corn tortillas
- 4 ounces grated extra-sharp Cheddar cheese
- 2 cups fresh salsa

Preheat oven to 350 degrees. In a medium saucepan, sauté onion and garlic in oil over medium heat until transparent and fragrant. Add chili powder, oregano, salt, cumin, red pepper flakes, and black-eyed peas. Reduce heat to medium low and cook for about 15 minutes. Add small amounts of water if the peas become too dry.

Remove from heat and place mixture in a large bowl. Mash the beans with a potato masher just enough to make them soft and stick together. You don't want to make a paste, but you don't want the peas to roll out when you fill the tortillas.

155

Warm tortillas in a toaster oven or over a hot comal, until pliable.

Spread each tortilla with about 2 tablespoons of peas and a sprinkle of cheese. Roll the tortilla. Place it seam-side down in a 9-by-13-baking pan. Repeat with remaining tortillas. Spoon salsa over tortillas. Top with remaining cheese. Bake 20 minutes, or until cheese is melted and enchiladas are thoroughly heated.

Nutrition per serving: 291 calories; 9 g Total Fat; 5 g saturated fat; 10 g protein; 40 g carbohydrates; 3 g dietary fiber; 0 mg cholesterol; 426 mg sodium.

Spanish Rice

This is a healthy version of my family's traditional recipe.

Makes 4 servings (serving = ½ cup)

- 1 cup long grain brown rice
- 2 tablespoons coconut oil
- 1 medium onion, minced
- 1 can (6 ounce) tomato sauce
- ½ cup water
- 1 cup fat-free chicken broth or vegetable broth
- 2 teaspoons ground cumin
- 1 small tomato, diced
- ½ cup fresh cilantro, chopped

Heat oil in a skillet over medium heat. Add the onion and sauté until translucent. Add the rice and stir constantly until the rice has browned and is slightly puffed. Add the tomato sauce, chicken broth, cumin, and diced tomato. Stir to mix thoroughly and bring to a boil. Let boil 5 minutes, stirring constantly. Reduce heat and simmer, covered, for 40-45 minutes.

Nutrition per serving: 218 calories; 8 g Total Fat; 6 g saturated fat; 4 g protein; 33 g carbohydrates; 1 g dietary fiber; 0 mg cholesterol; 29 mg sodium.

Southwestern Chick Pea Stew

Garbanzos, also called chick-peas, are unique round beans with a nice nutty taste.

Makes 6 servings (serving = ½ cup)

- 2 tablespoons coconut oil
- 2 small onions, chopped
- 6 cloves fresh garlic, minced
- 2 cans (15 ounce) garbanzo beans, rinsed and drained
- 1 can (14 ounce) stewed tomatoes, chopped (reserve the liquid)
- ½ teaspoon dried basil
- ½ teaspoon ground cumin
- 2 teaspoons chili powder
- ½ teaspoon dried Mexican oregano
- 1 tablespoon fresh cilantro, chopped

Heat the oil in a large, deep pan over medium heat. Sauté the onions until they are very tender. Add the garlic, stirring the mixture until the onions turn golden. Add the garbanzos, tomatoes (and their liquid), basil, chili powder, oregano, cilantro, and cumin. Cover and simmer over low heat for 25 minutes until thick.

Serve as is or over freshly cooked Spanish rice.

Nutrition per serving: 222 calories; 7 g Total Fat; 4 g saturated fat; 9 g protein; 32 g carbohydrates; 8 g dietary fiber; 0 mg cholesterol; 21 mg sodium.

Roasted Tomatillo Salsa

Tomatillos are small green fruits with a papery outer skin. A relative of the tomato family, tomatillos provide the tart flavor in many Mexican green sauces and salsas.

Makes 2 cups (serving = ½ cup)

- 1 pound (7 medium) tomatillos, husked and rinsed
- 4 to 5 fresh serrano chilies, stemmed
- 1 small white onion, sliced ¼ inch thick
- 6 garlic cloves, peeled
- ½ cup water or more
- 1/3 cup fresh cilantro
- 1 teaspoon sea salt
- 3 drops liquid stevia or to taste

Heat the broiler. Lay the whole tomatillos and serranos on a broiler pan or baking sheet. Set the pan 4 inches below the broiler and let roast until the tomatillos are softened and splotchy black in places, about 5 minutes. They should change from light bright green to olive green on the top side. With a pair of tongs, flip over the tomatillos and chilies and roast the other side for an additional 4 to 5 minutes. Set aside to cool.

Preheat oven to 425 degrees. Separate the onion into rings. On another pan or baking sheet, mix the onion and garlic cloves. Roast in oven for about 15 minutes, stirring every few minutes, until the onions are richly browned, wilted and slightly charred on some of the edges. The garlic should be soft and browned in spots. Remove from the oven and cool to room temperature.

159

In a food processor, pulse the onions, garlic and serranos until finely chopped, scraping sides as needed. Scoop into a large bowl. Without washing the processor, coarsely puree the tomatillos; no need to peel off the darkened skin or to cut out their cores. Stir them into the chilies, adding enough water to give the salsa an easily spoonable consistency. Stir in cilantro.

Taste the salsa and season it with salt to taste. Taste again and add just enough stevia to take the edge off the bright tanginess of the tomatillos.

Nutrition per serving: 88 calories; 0 g Total Fat; 0 g saturated fat; 3 g protein; 17 g carbohydrates; 2 g dietary fiber; 0 mg cholesterol; 583 mg sodium.

Healthful Snack Ideas

Forget dropping coins in a vending machine when you're hungry for a snack. These are some of my favorite things to munch on when I get a snack attack.

Sweet 'n Spicy Mixed Nuts

These nuts have a unique flavor and are great for snacks at any time. Keep some in the car for emergency snack attacks!

Makes 1 pound, about 16 servings
(serving = 1 ounce, about ¼ cup)

- ½ pound raw almonds
- ½ pound raw cashews
- 2 tablespoons butter
- ¼ teaspoon cayenne pepper
- 1/8 cup Rapadura sugar or Sucanat
- 3 drops liquid stevia extract
- a few dashes of sea salt

Preheat oven to 250 degrees. In a large bowl, mix together the raw almonds and raw cashews. Pour the nuts into a skillet at medium high heat for a few minutes. Toast the nuts until slightly brown, stirring frequently to get all nuts toasted. Remove when brown and pour back into the large bowl.

Melt the butter in the same skillet over medium low heat. Add the Rapadura or Sucanat and stevia. Stir until the Rapadura or Sucanat is melted and blended with the butter. Add the cayenne pepper and a few dashes of sea salt to the butter mixture. Pour butter mixture over the nuts and mix well with a spoon, making sure all of the nuts get covered.

Spread the nuts evenly onto a baking sheet and roast at 250 degrees for 30 minutes. Remove from the oven and cool before placing in a covered container such as a Tupperware.

Nutrition per serving: 212 calories; 16 g Total Fat; 2 g saturated fat; 7 g protein; 9 g carbohydrates; 2.5 g dietary fiber; 4 mg cholesterol; 72 mg sodium.

Apple and Almond Butter

Great for the kids or for a mid-morning energy boost.

Makes 1 serving

- 1 apple, sliced (preferably organic)
- 1 tablespoon natural almond butter

Slice up the apple (preferably organic) and spread some natural almond butter on the slices.

Nutrition per serving: 212 calories; 8 g Total Fat; 0 g saturated fat; 4 g protein; 33 g carbohydrates; 5 g dietary fiber; 0 mg cholesterol; 0 mg sodium.

Raw Trail Mix

Make your own Trail Mix and you avoid the sugar, candy and the hydrogenated oils that are in many commercially available mixes. Great for those times when you're hungry and on the run. Keep a baggie in your car or office!

Makes 24 servings (serving = ¼ cup)

- 1 cup raw almonds
- 1 cup raw cashews
- 1 cup raw pecans
- 1 cup raw walnuts
- 1 cup raisins
- ½ cup unsweetened coconut flakes

Mix ingredients together in a large bowl. Measure out ¼ cup of the mixture and place into individual snack size baggies. This is a great snack to grab and go.

Nutrition per serving: 165 calories; 12 g Total Fat; 2 g saturated fat; 4 g protein; 9 g carbohydrates; 2 g dietary fiber; 0 mg cholesterol; 2 mg sodium.

Banana, Peanut Butter and Brown Rice Cakes

These fun snacks provide substantial and sustained energy.

Makes 1 serving

- 1 small banana, sliced
- 1 tablespoon natural peanut butter
- 1 brown rice cake

Spread peanut butter on rice cake and top with banana slices – great for a mid-afternoon snack.

Nutrition per serving: 242 calories; 8 g Total Fat; 1 g saturated fat; 6 g protein; 34 g carbohydrates; 2 g dietary fiber; 0 mg cholesterol; 80 mg sodium.

Tasteful Appetizer Spread

Great for guests and so easy to create!

Makes 20 servings

- 1 (5 ounce log) Goat cheese
- 1 box Ak Mak crackers or whole wheat crackers
- 20 dried apricot halves, unsulphured
- ¼ pound raw almonds
- ¼ pound raw cashews
- ¼ pound raw walnuts

Arrange ingredients on platter for guests to enjoy before dinner. Also makes for a filling snack.

Nutrition per serving: 158 calories; 12 g Total Fat; 2.5 g saturated fat; 5 g protein; 8 g carbohydrates; 1 g dietary fiber; 6 mg cholesterol; 64 mg sodium.

Plan-D Flourless Muffins™ a la Mode

Some of our friends have discovered this to be a great desert-like treat!

Makes 1 serving (serving = 1 muffin and ½ cup yogurt)

- Plan-D Flourless Muffin (either buy them or make them yourself (see index)
- 1/2 cup Easy Vanilla Yogurt (see index) or 2 Tablespoons Real Deal Whipped Cream (see index)

Warm the muffin in an oven or toaster oven. Place in a bowl and top with Easy Vanilla Yogurt or Real Deal Whipped Cream.

Nutrition per serving: 186 calories; 5 g Total Fat; 0 g saturated fat; 10 g protein; 26 g carbohydrates; 4 g dietary fiber; 0 mg cholesterol; 260 mg sodium.

Vegetable Spread

Another great appetizer for guests to enjoy!

Makes 5 servings (serving = 1 cup veggies plus ½ cup hummus)

- 1 cup baby carrots
- 1 cup celery stalks, cut into 1 inch segments
- 1 Bell pepper, sliced into thick strips
- 1 cup broccoli florets
- 1 cup Cauliflower florets
- 2 ½ cups Hummus

Place vegetables on plate with hummus. Hummus is made from ground garbanzo beans, so it's loaded with fiber. It's also good spread on brown rice cakes or Ak Mak crackers. Buy hummus already made or make your own

Nutrition per serving: 225 calories; 7 g Total Fat; <1 g saturated fat; 8 g protein; 33 g carbohydrates; 3 g dietary fiber; 0 mg cholesterol; 635 mg sodium.

Sweet Potato Hummus

Great for an everyday appetizer.

Makes 6 servings (serving = ½ cup)

- 1 pound sweet potatoes
- 1 teaspoon cumin seeds, crushed
- 1 large lemon, juiced
- 1 teaspoon salt
- ¼ teaspoon cayenne pepper
- 1/8 teaspoon black pepper
- 1 tablespoon tahini (sesame seed paste, available in gourmet food stores)
- 1 tablespoon olive oil
- zest of 1 orange

Create Baked Sweet Potatoes (see index). Allow them to cool, then remove and discard the skins. Toast cumin seeds in a skillet on low heat, then crush with a mortar and pestle or by smashing between a saucepan and cutting board.

Add all ingredients to food processor and blend until smooth and creamy.

Nutrition per serving: 118 calories; 4 g Total Fat; <1 g saturated fat; 2 g protein; 19 g carbohydrates; 1 g dietary fiber; 0 mg cholesterol; 385 mg sodium.

Tasty Beverages

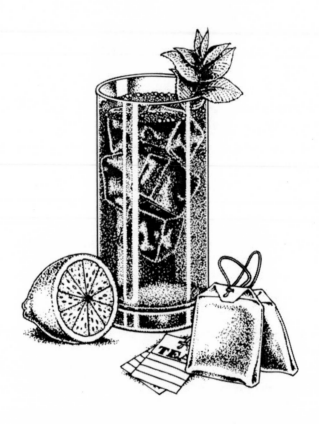

Beverages should be just as healthful as our food. These flavorful drinks provide vitamins and nutrients.

Warm Lemon Water

Start your morning with lemon water, for it cleanses and supports your body's main fat-burning organ – the liver. Some of my nutrition students have discovered this beverage has replaced their need for coffee in the morning.

Makes 1 serving

- 8 - 16 ounces of warm water
- juice from 1/2 fresh squeezed lemon

Add the juice to water. Drink before breakfast to establish movement of your lymphatic system before you start your day. Water should be the temperature of a cup of hot tea. Use only fresh lemon juice.

Nutrition per serving: 11 calories; 0 g Total Fat; 0 g saturated fat; 0 g protein; 3 g carbohydrates; 0 g dietary fiber; 0 mg cholesterol; 1 mg sodium.

Ice Cold Lemonade

Great for those hot summer days!

Makes 2 quarts (serving = 1 cup)

- 2 quarts water
- 8 fresh lemons
- 1 teaspoon liquid Stevia extract, or to taste

Fill a 2 quart pitcher with water. Squeeze the juice from the lemons into the water. Add stevia to taste. Serve over ice.

Nutrition per serving: 22 calories; 0 g Total Fat; 0 g saturated fat; 0 g protein; 5 g carbohydrates; 0 g dietary fiber; 0 mg cholesterol; 1 mg sodium.

Ginger Ale

Fresh ginger helps improve digestion!

Makes 1 serving

- 2 teaspoons fresh ginger, peeled and grated
- 1 tablespoon fresh squeezed lemon or lime juice
- 16 ounces sparkling water, unflavored
- 2-3 drops liquid stevia extract, or to taste

Place the lemon or lime juice in a glass and add the ginger. Stir together. Add the sparkling water and stevia. Stir again. Add ice cubes and drink immediately.

Nutrition per serving: 8 calories; 0 g Total Fat; 0 g saturated fat; 0 g protein; 2 g carbohydrates; 0 g dietary fiber; 0 mg cholesterol; 1 mg sodium.

Hot "Cocoa"

Great for cold mornings or cold evenings.

Makes 1 serving

- 1 cup soy milk, almond milk, rice milk, or low-fat cow's milk
- 1 teaspoon pure vanilla extract
- 3 drops liquid Stevia extract, or to taste
- 1 teaspoon unsweetened carob powder
- ¼ teaspoon cardamom
- ¼ teaspoon cinnamon

Heat the milk in a saucepan over medium heat, but do not boil. Add carob powder, stevia, and spices. Stir until thoroughly mixed. Transfer to a mug and drink immediately.

Nutrition per serving: 50 calories; 3 g Total Fat; 0 g saturated fat; 1 g protein; 6 g carbohydrates; 0 g dietary fiber; 0 mg cholesterol; 180 mg sodium.

Cranberry Spritzer

Diet sodas contain harmful phosphates and artificial sweeteners. This spritzer is a healthy alternative for those who enjoy bubbly drinks.

Makes 1 serving

- 1 fluid ounce unsweetened cranberry juice*
- 16 ounces sparkling water, unflavored
- 2-3 drops liquid stevia extract, or to taste

Fill a glass with ice. Pour in sparkling water, cranberry juice, and stevia. Stir and enjoy with a straw!

*More on cranberry juice:

It's very important to buy only <u>unsweetened</u> cranberry juice—not the no-sugar added kind. Such brands may contain high fructose corn syrup or artificial sweeteners. Unsweetened cranberry juice can be purchased from natural food stores.

Nutrition per serving: 7 calories; 0 g Total Fat; 0 g saturated fat; 0 g protein; 2 g carbohydrates; 0 g dietary fiber; 0 mg cholesterol; 21 mg sodium.

Allowable Indulgences

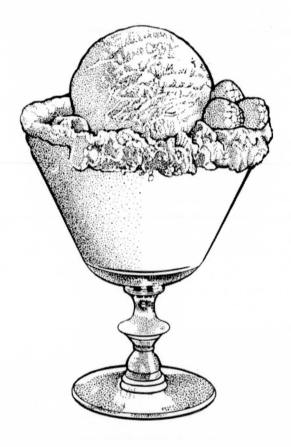

Who says dessert can't be healthy? These treats are so delicious, people can't believe they don't have sugar in them. A word of caution: it's very important to know your own limits when it comes to sweet treats.

M and G's Rapadura Vanilla Ice Cream

Rapadura is an unrefined sugar that can almost be considered a whole food. It is processed by grinding up the whole natural sugar cane and evaporating off the water. The remaining coarse, golden grain retains all of the essential vitamins, minerals, fiber and nutrients contained in the natural sugar cane. Use the stevia for a completely sugar-free version.

Makes 3-4 cups (serving = ½ cup)

- 3 egg yolks
- ½ cup Rapadura or ½ teaspoon bulk stevia powder
- ¼ real vanilla bean
- 1 cup half and half, preferably organic
- 2 cups lite coconut milk
- ½ teaspoon sea salt

Put egg yolks, half and half, Rapadura, salt and ¼ real vanilla bean (split) in a sauce pan. Place on medium heat just till bubbles form. Remove from heat and fish out the vanilla pod and scrape out the seeds into the mixture. The more seeds you get, the more vanilla flavor. Discard the pod. Cool to room temperature.

Add coconut milk and place in an ice cream maker. If you don't have an ice cream maker, you can place the mixture into a covered bowl and put it in the freezer. However, you must stir every 15 minutes and return to the freezer or it will be icy.

Nutrition per serving: 146 calories; 9 g Total Fat; 6 g saturated fat; 2 g protein; 14 g carbohydrates; 0 g dietary fiber; 87 mg cholesterol; 179 mg sodium.

Special thanks to Marcy Neves and Gretchen Maynard, two of my nutrition students, for contributing this recipe.

Allowable Sin™

These treats are loaded with protein, good fat, and fiber. Not your ordinary chocolate bar. Beware, these treats are addicting!

Makes 32 pieces (serving = 1 piece)

- 1 scoop whey protein powder, vanilla flavored (stevia sweetened only)
- 2 tablespoons unsweetened carob powder
- ¼ cup unsweetened dried coconut flakes (preferably organic and unsulfured)
- ¼ cup raw cashews, chopped
- ¼ cup raw almonds, chopped
- ¼ cup raisins or chopped dates
- ½ cup chunky natural peanut butter
- 2 ounces unsweetened baker's chocolate
- ½ to 1 teaspoon stevia extract, or to taste
- ¼ cup unrefined coconut oil, liquid at room temperature
- 1 teaspoon pure vanilla extract
- 32 mini size paper baking cups (cupcake liners), about the size of truffles

Chop the baker's chocolate into small pieces.

Place the coconut oil in a small saucepan and add the chopped chocolate. Place the pan over a low heat and allow the chocolate to melt into the coconut oil. Stir frequently with a rubber spatula. When the chocolate is completely melted, remove from heat and set aside.

179

In a large bowl, combine the protein powder, carob or cocoa powder, coconut, chopped almonds, chopped cashews, chopped dates or raisins, and shredded coconut. Mix together well with a spoon. Add in the peanut butter and mix thoroughly. At this point the mixture should be somewhat crumbly.

Add the vanilla extract and the stevia to the melted chocolate mixture in the saucepan and stir to mix thoroughly. Transfer the melted chocolate mixture to the bowl, using the rubber spatula to scrape out the saucepan.

Stir the mixture thoroughly to combine. Use a small measuring spoon, such as a teaspoon, to scoop and fill the baking cups with the chocolate mixture. Put them in a baking dish or other large flat container and place in the freezer until the truffles harden, about 30 minutes. Store in the freezer until ready to eat.

Note: when frozen, the paper cup peels off easily and you will have a chocolate delight that resembles a mini Reese's Peanut Butter Cup (without the sugar and trans-fats)!

Nutrition per serving: 80 calories; 6 g Total Fat; 3 g saturated fat; 3 g protein; 3 g carbohydrates; 1 g dietary fiber; 0 mg cholesterol; 8 mg sodium.

Sunflower-Almond-Sesame Tahini Logs

The flavors of sesame, tahini and almonds complement each other in a truly magnificent way.

Makes 1 dozen logs

- 1 cup sunflower seed meal, ground fresh
- ½ cup tahini
- ¼ cup raw unfiltered honey
- ¼ cup raw almonds, ground into fine powder
- 1 cup dates, chopped
- ½ cup unsweetened ground coconut
- Whole raw almonds

Combine ingredients in order given. Mix thoroughly. Separate mixture into two portions; roll into logs. Wrap each mixture in wax paper and store in refrigerator. When chilled, remove and cut into half inch pieces. Press a whole almond on each piece for eye appeal.

Nutrition per serving: 248 calories; 16 g Total Fat; 4 g saturated fat; 5 g protein; 22 g carbohydrates; 2 g dietary fiber; 0 mg cholesterol; 2 mg sodium.

High Protein Granola Bars

Warning! These bars are extremely delicious and may require many friends to help you eat them. Don't stay home alone with a batch in the freezer!

Makes one 9 ½ x 11" baking dish, cut into bars the size of your preference (for purposes of nutrition per serving, the pan was cut into 24 bars)

Dry Ingredients:
- 2 cups oatmeal
- ½ cup whey protein powder, vanilla flavored (stevia sweetened only)
- 2 tablespoons carob powder (optional)
- ½ cup pepitas, lightly toasted
- ¼ cup sesame seeds, lightly toasted
- 1 cup raw cashews, chopped
- 1 cup raw almonds, chopped
- 2 tablespoons flaxseeds, whole or ground
- 2/3 cup unsweetened coconut flakes
- ½ cup raisins

Wet Ingredients:
- ½ cup coconut oil (liquid at room temperature)
- 2 teaspoons pure vanilla extract
- ½ cup raw unfiltered honey or brown rice syrup
- ½ cup natural peanut butter

In a large bowl, combine the dry ingredients. Mix well. In a separate bowl, add vanilla to the coconut oil and whisk together, mixing well. Add in honey or brown rice syrup.

Add in peanut butter and whisk until the mixture is uniform in texture. Add the wet ingredients to the dry ingredients with a large spoon. Stir until all the dry ingredients are coated with the wet, mixing thoroughly. Transfer the mixture to a 9½ X 11 glass baking dish. Spread evenly and pat down. Cover the pan with plastic wrap and refrigerate several hours or overnight. To serve, slice into bars. Bars are best kept in the refrigerator until ready to be served.

Nutrition per serving: 255 calories; 17 g Total Fat; 7 g saturated fat; 8 g protein; 18 g carbohydrates; 1 g dietary fiber; 0 mg cholesterol; 42 mg sodium

Date-Walnut Pie Crust

This is a delicious, flourless, pie crust.

Makes 1 pie crust (cut into 10 pieces, serving = 1 piece)

- 1 pound soft dates, pitted
- ½ pound walnuts, ground to flour consistency
- ¾ cup shredded organic unsweetened coconut

Grind walnuts to flour consistency by placing in a food processor or coffee grinder. Set aside. Clean the food processor to use for the dates. Place the dates in a food processor and pulse to make a paste. Transfer date paste to a mixing bowl, add ground walnuts and coconut and knead together forming a "dough". Press into a 10-inch pie plate. Refrigerate to harden. Fill with your favorite pie filling.

Nutrition per serving: 343 calories; 19 g Total Fat; 5 g saturated fat; 5 g protein; 39 g carbohydrates; 3 g dietary fiber; 0 mg cholesterol; 6 mg sodium

Organic Apple Delight

Conventionally grown apples may have a high amount of pesticide residue on them. You should choose organic whenever possible. I often have this dish with my muffins.

Makes 6 servings (serving = ½ cup)

- 3 medium size organic apples, sliced into thin pieces (choose a variety of sweet and/or tart apples)
- Fresh squeezed juice from 1 small organic lemon
- Small piece of lemon rind, finely chopped
- ¼ cup water
- ½ cup organic raisins or ½ cup chopped organic medjool dates
- Small amount of raw unfiltered organic honey, to taste
- 1 teaspoon cinnamon
- 1 teaspoon pumpkin pie spice (see recipe on next page)
- 3 tablespoons ground raw organic almonds

Core apples and slice into thin pieces. Place apples, lemon juice, finely chopped lemon rind and water in a saucepan. Stir and cook over medium high heat.

When mixture starts to bubble, lower the heat. Add honey, cinnamon, pumpkin pie spice, ground almonds, and raisins as you stir mixture. Continue cooking at low heat for approximately 15 to 20 minutes or until mixture is soft enough to mash with a potato masher. Cover and let cool on stove top. Serve warm with vanilla yogurt or a muffin.

Nutrition per serving: 131 calories; 5 g Total Fat; 0 g saturated fat; 1.5 g protein; 20 g carbohydrates; 2 g dietary fiber; 0 mg cholesterol; 1 mg sodium

Organic Pumpkin Pie

This is the most wholesome pie you've ever tasted. Your holiday guests will never know it's organic and healthy!

Makes one 9-inch pie (8 servings per pie, serving = 1/8 pie)

- 1 can (15 ounce) organic canned pumpkin or 2 cups cooked organic pumpkin
- 2 large eggs
- ¾ cup coconut milk
- ¾ cup Rapadura sugar or Sucanat
- 1 ½ teaspoons ground cinnamon
- ¾ teaspoon ground ginger
- ¼ teaspoon ground cloves
- ½ teaspoon sea salt
- 1 unbaked 9-inch deep dish whole wheat pie crust

Preheat oven to 425 degrees. Mix Rapadura or Sucanat, cinnamon, ginger, cloves, and salt in a small bowl. In a separate large bowl, beat eggs. Stir in the pumpkin and then add in the sugar-spice mixture. Gradually stir in the coconut milk and mix until well blended.

Pour into the unbaked pie shell. Bake in the preheated oven at 425 degrees for 15 minutes, then reduce oven temperature to 350 degrees and bake for an additional 40 to 50 minutes or until a knife inserted into the center comes out clean. Cool on a wire rack for 2 hours. Immediately serve or refrigerate. Top with Real Deal Whipped Cream, see recipe p. xx)

Nutrition per serving: 172 calories; 7 g Total Fat; 4 g saturated fat; 3 g protein; 26 g carbohydrates; 1 g dietary fiber; 74 mg cholesterol; 189 mg sodium

Araby's Tropical Dream Pops

This is a fun way to chill out on a hot day.

Makes 6 pops (serving = 1 pop)

- 2 cups plain nonfat yogurt, preferably organic
- ½ can (4 ounce) crushed pineapple, in its own juice
- 1 ripe banana, mashed
- ½ cup dried unsweetened coconut, shredded
- ¼ to ½ teaspoon liquid stevia, to taste
- Dixie paper cups and popsicle sticks

Place all ingredients into a blender or food processor and blend until smooth. Spoon yogurt mixture into paper cups. Freeze for 45 minutes or until the mixture starts to thicken. Place wooden sticks into cups and freeze at least 4 hours. Eat frozen, and eat them fast!

Special thanks goes to Araby Cash, my friend, for her contribution to this recipe.

Nutrition per serving: 115 calories; 4 g Total Fat; 4 g saturated fat; 4 g protein; 14 g carbohydrates; 0.5 g dietary fiber; 0 mg cholesterol; 56 mg sodium

Gelatin Fruit Salad

This refreshing fruit salad is great for breakfast, snacks or dessert!

Makes 4 servings (serving = 1 cup)

- 1 envelope Knox unflavored gelatin
- ½ cup boiling water
- one 6 ounce can pineapple juice
- one 8 ounce can pineapple chunks** (unsweetened, in its own juice)
- 1 tablespoon lemon juice
- 1 cup sliced strawberries
- 1 large banana, sliced
- ½ cup dried unsweetened coconut flakes (unsulfured and preferably organic)

In a medium bowl, add gelatin to boiling water and stir until dissolved. Drain the juice from the can of pineapple chunks and add it to the gelatin. Add the 6 ounce can of pineapple juice and the lemon juice and stir.

Add the pineapple chunks, strawberries, and banana slices and stir. Sprinkle the top with unsweetened coconut. Chill until set, at least 4 hours. Serve with Vanilla Yogurt (see index).

**Note: Do not use fresh pineapple for this salad. There are enzymes in fresh pineapple that interfere with the "geling" properties of gelatin and it won't gel properly.

Nutrition per serving: 193 calories; 7 g Total Fat; 6 g saturated fat; 5 g protein; 28 g carbohydrates; 1 g dietary fiber; 0 mg cholesterol; 9 mg sodium.

Rich Mocha Tofu Mousse

Tastes just like the real thing, only it's much better for you! For this recipe, it is very important to use <u>silken</u> tofu, and it must be the <u>extra-firm</u> variety. Silken tofu is much creamier in it's texture. Regular tofu will not work—you will be very disappointed in how this recipe turns out if you don't use silken tofu!

Makes 6 servings (serving = ½ cup)

- 1 Package (12.3 ounce) extra-firm, silken tofu (shelf stable Mori-Nu brand preferred)
- 2 ounces unsweetened baker's chocolate
- 1/4 cup unsweetened carob powder
- 1 tablespoon instant espresso or coffee powder
- ½ teaspoon pure vanilla extract
- ¼ teaspoon or more liquid stevia, to taste

Drain the tofu in a colander for about 10 minutes. Meanwhile, chop the chocolate into small pieces. Melt the chocolate.

Place the tofu in a food processor or blender. Puree until creamy, about 30 seconds, scraping down the bowl once or twice. Fold in the carob powder and espresso powder. Puree until well blended, scraping down the bowl as needed. Add the vanilla, stevia, and melted chocolate. Puree until smooth.

Transfer to individual dishes or a large bowl. Cover and chill several hours or overnight.

To dress up the mousse, serve it in individual goblets. Garnish with fresh raspberries and a sprig of mint.

Nutrition per serving: 183 calories; 9 g Total Fat; 3 g saturated fat; 17 g protein; 12 g carbohydrates; 1 g dietary fiber; 0 mg cholesterol; 147 mg sodium.

Easy Vanilla Yogurt

If plain yogurt is too sour for your palate, try this lightly sweet variety. All vanilla extracts are not created equal. Beware of vanilla extracts that contain corn syrup.

Makes 1 serving

- 1 cup non-fat plain yogurt, organic preferred
- 1 teaspoon pure vanilla extract
- Liquid stevia to taste
- 1 teaspoon ground cinnamon (optional)

Place all ingredients in a bowl and stir until vanilla extract has been thoroughly mixed in and you no longer see its color. Enjoy immediately!

Nutrition per serving: 120 calories; 0 g Total Fat; 0 g saturated fat; 11 g protein; 19 g carbohydrates; 0 g dietary fiber; 0 mg cholesterol; 160 mg sodium.

Baked Apples

Great for a snack or dessert, but also a very satisfying breakfast.

Makes 4 servings

- 4 organic apples, preferably red
- ½ chopped dates
- ¼ cup chopped pecans or walnuts
- 2 tablespoons fresh lemon juice
- 1 teaspoon ground cinnamon
- 1 cup fat-free plain or vanilla yogurt (optional)

Preheat oven to 350°F. Using a corer or paring knife, remove core from each apple without cutting through the bottom. Make the hole 1 inch larger in diameter to accommodate the filling. Combine the dates, lemon juice and cinnamon in a small bowl, and spoon this mixture into the apples. Place in an 8-inch baking pan. Fill the pan halfway with water and bake until soft, 30 to 35 minutes. Serve warm with ¼ cup yogurt on top of each apple.

Nutrition per serving:

Baked Apple Only: 192 calories; 5 g Total Fat; 0 g saturated fat; 2 g protein; 34 g carbohydrates; 5 g dietary fiber; 0 mg cholesterol; 1 mg sodium.

With Yogurt: 222 calories; 5 g Total Fat; 0 g saturated fat; 4 g protein; 39 g carbohydrates; 5 g dietary fiber; 0 mg cholesterol; 41 mg sodium.

Real Deal Whipped Cream

Fat-free and sugar-free non-dairy whipped cream substitutes are loaded with artificial chemical ingredients. There's no healthy substitute for real cream, but there is a substitute for sugar!

Makes 2 cups

- 1 pint whipping cream, preferably organic
- 1/8 teaspoon liquid stevia

Chill a large mixing bowl in the freezer for 10 minutes. Remove the bowl from the freezer and pour the whipping cream into it. Beat with an electric mixer until the cream begins to thicken. Add the stevia slowly, ensuring that it gets mixed in. Continue beating until stiff peaks form.
Use immediately. Remainder can be saved in an airtight container for 3-4 days.

Nutrition per serving: 54 calories; 6 g Total Fat; 4 g saturated fat; 0 g protein; 0 g carbohydrates; 0 g dietary fiber; 25 mg cholesterol; 0 mg sodium.

Bibliography

- Appleton, Nancy. *Lick the Sugar Habit*. Avery Publishing Company, 1996.
- Bragg, Paul, N.D., Ph.D. and Bragg, Patricia N.D., Ph.D. *Apple Cider Vinegar Health System*, Health Science.
- Buetler, Jade, R.R.T., R.C.P. *Weight Loss with Flaxseed, the Non-fat Fat*, Health Perspectives.
- *Complex Carbohydrates*, Weight-Loss.co.uk, retrieved from the World Wide Web, 2002.
- *Food For Life*. http://www.mybloodsugar.net/foodforlife.htm, retrieved from the World Wide Web, 2005.
- Fuhrman, Joel. M.D. *Eat to Live*. Little, Brown and Company, 2003.
- Gates, Donna and Sahelian, Ray M.D. *The Stevia Cookbook*. Avery Publishing Company, 1999.
- Gittleman, Anne Louise, M.S., C.N.S. *The Fat Flush Plan*, McGraw-Hill, 2002.
- Grieger, Lynn, R.D., C.D.E. *Simple vs. Complex Carbohydrates*. Ivillage.co.uk, retrieved from the World Wide Web, 2002.
- Holzapfel, Cynthia. *Apple Cider Vinegar For Weight Loss and Good Health*, Healthy Living Publications, 2002.
- Liebman, Bonnie. *Healthful Whole Grains*. Center for Science in the Public Interest Nutrition Action Newsletter, www.cspinet.org/nah/wwheat.html, retrieved from the World Wide Web, 2005.
- London, Jan. *Coconut Cuisine Featuring Stevia*, J. L. Books, 2004.
- McCaleb Herb Research Foundation. *Stevia Leaf - Too Good To Be Legal?*, www.anniesappleseedproject,org, retrieved from the World Wide Web, 2005.
- McCullogh, Fran. *The Good Fat Cookbook*, Scribner, 2003.
- *Refined Carbohydrates are to Blame for Skyrocketing Chronic Disease, Not Just Obesity*. News Target Network, retrieved from the World Wide Web, 2004.
- Rodio, Mary, Dr. *Refined Food: Even the Bugs Won't Eat It*. Dentizyme.com, retrieved from the World Wide Web, 2002.
- Spreen, A.N., M.D. *Everything You Ever Wanted to Know About Refined Carbohydrates*. Ivillage.com, retrieved from the World Wide Web, 2002.
- Stinton, Maxine. *Breads, Cereals and Potatoes*. BBC.co.uk, retrieved from the World Wide Web, 2002.

Index

195

Breinigsville, PA USA
01 September 2009
223368BV00001B/66/P